Medical Instrumentation for Nurses and Allied Health-Care Professionals

Richard Aston, Ph.D., P.E.

East Tennessee State University
Johnson City, Tennessee

Katherine Kay Brown, M.S.N., R.N., C.C.R.N.

Allegheny General Hospital
Pittsburgh, Pennsylvania

LaRoche College
Pittsburgh, Pennsylvania

JONES AND BARTLETT PUBLISHERS
BOSTON   LONDON

Editorial, Sales, and Customer Service Offices
Jones and Bartlett Publishers
One Exeter Plaza
Boston, MA 02116
1-800-832-0034
1-617-859-3900

Jones and Bartlett Publishers International
P.O. Box 1498
London W6 7RS
England

Library of Congress Cataloging-in-Publication Data
Aston, Richard.
    Medical instrumentation for nurses and allied health-care
professionals / Richard Aston, Katherine Kay Brown.
        p.   cm.
    Includes bibliographical references and index.
    ISBN 0–86720–688–8
    1. Medical instruments and apparatus.   2. Medical technology.
3. Nursing.   I. Brown, Katherine Kay.   II. Title.
[DNLM: 1. Equipment and Supplies, Hospital.   2. Equipment Safety.
WX 147   1994]
R856.A798   1994
610'.28—dc20
DNLM/DLC
for Library of Congress   94–5992
                                                              CIP

Acquisitions Editor: Jan Wall
Production Editor: Anne Noonan
Manufacturing Buyer: Dana L. Cerrito
Design: Linda Zuk, WordCrafters Editorial Services, Inc.
Editorial Production: WordCrafters Editorial Services, Inc.
Illustrations: Freehold Studio
Typesetting: A & B Typesetters, Inc.
Cover Design: Hannus Design Associates
Printing and Binding: Braun-Brumfield, Inc.
Cover Printing: New England Book Components, Inc.

Printed in the United States of America

97 96 95 94   10 9 8 7 6 5 4 3 2 1

To Marcia,
Edward,
William
and Vince

Contents

Chapter 4
THE ELECTROCARDIOGRAPH
Richard Aston and *Jean C. Hemphill*

Chapter 5
MICROPROCESSOR-BASED EQUIPMENT
Richard Aston

Chapter 8
LASERS AND SURGICAL DEVICES   185
Richard Aston

Chapter 9
INTRAVENOUS PUMPS AND CATHETERS   225
Richard Aston, Katherine K. Brown, and *Carol Wysowski*

Chapter 10
VENTILATORS AND PULMONARY
FUNCTION MONITORING   271

Jean C. Hemphill and *Richard Aston*

Preface

This book is intended to increase the understanding of medical instrumentation for health-care providers. It is consistent with the background of the nurse and offers answers to the serious questions nurses may have about the equipment on and in their patients. Therefore, the emphasis is on patient-care equipment, such as defibrillators, intravenous (IV) pumps, pacemakers, ventilators, and diagnostic equipment.

The health-care provider, with respect to medical instrumentation, is patient oriented. This gives rise to a need for understanding equipment safety and developing safe operating procedures. The responsibility for preventative maintenance, troubleshooting, and the repair of equipment implanted in or attached to the patient often falls to the nurse when specialists such as therapists or biomedical engineering technologists (BMETs) are not immediately available. In some cases, the BMET doesn't have the background to understand the patient–machine interface and needs to work with the nurse to solve an equipment problem. This book will also help the BMET become more effective in dealing with equipment problems in the hospital or clinic.

The special needs of the health-care provider are served by this book through extensive discussions of the medical indications for use of the equipment. Also, in order to respond immediately to patient symptoms, the medical complications that can evolve from equipment use need to be understood.

The number of new and complicated instruments that have been introduced into medical/surgical nursing in recent years is large. This equipment, such as external pacemakers, defibrillators, central venous catheters, and ventilators, is complicated and can be dangerous to the patient if not handled properly. Because this equipment has become microprocessor based, modes of operation, along with confusing acronyms, have proliferated. This book will help clarify this situation for the health-care professional.

The personal satisfaction that the professional gains from using this book is the knowledge that the patient's safety and comfort may be increased, along with the accuracy of the diagnostic data or applied therapy. Study of this book may also help the professional's career by providing preparation for more interesting, highly technical assignments, which could lead to professional advancement.

The need for improvements in undergraduate college education on medical instrumentation for nurses has been studied extensively over the past decade by June Abbey, Ph.D., R.N. Indeed, her work provided the single most important inspiration for the undertaking of this project. Those who use the Abbey/Shepherd model for device education will find the materials necessary for most of its components in this text.

The points made about the equipment described in this text include:

- Information processing.
- Instrumentation principles.
- Patient–machine interface.
- Medical indications for use.
- Medical complications.
- Operating procedures.

The emphasis is on the generic device, developing a holistic perspective, and giving the user the proper background for understanding the equipment manuals supplied by the manufacturers, which will give specific operating and troubleshooting information for the devices they manufacture.

The first three chapters present the basic background information necessary to understand the issues surrounding hospital-based equipment. In Chapter 1, both the historical approach and the theoretical approach based on physical laws are given. Chapter 2 discusses the specific issue of hospital equipment safety. And in Chapter 3, the way machines process physiological parameters is discussed. Chapters 4 and 5 discuss diagnostic monitors and information processing with microprocessors.

The remaining half of the book answers the specific questions health-care providers have about therapeutic equipment, including internal and external pacemakers and defibrillators, IV pumps and catheters, and ventilators and surgical devices. These are treated in terms of information processing, principles of operation, medical indications for use, and complications. Guidelines are also developed for instructing the patient who uses the equipment.

The information and recommendations contained in this book are not intended for specific applications, but are of a general educational nature. The author and publisher disclaim liability of any kind arising as a result of application of the subject matter of this book.

Acknowledgments

This book would not have been possible without the work of those listed in the references. Early supporters of this project include Marcia H. Aston, wife and librarian at Wilkes-Barre General Hospital. The librarians at Mercy Hospital, Wilkes-Barre, Barbara Nanstiel and Joan Zafia, contributed generously to this project. The help of Dr. Ann Kolanowski, chairperson of Nursing at Wilkes University, Diana Morgan, M.S., R.N., at Wilkes-Barre General Hospital, and Dr. Wayne Andrews at East Tennessee State University greatly facilitated the making of the collaboration between biomedical engineering and nursing that makes this project unique.

Contributors

Richard Aston, Ph.D., P.E.
East Tennessee State University
Johnson City, TN

Katherine Kay Brown, M.S.N., R.N., C.C.R.N.
Allegheny General Hospital
Pittsburgh, PA

LaRoche College
Pittsburgh, PA

Jean Croce Hemphill, M.S.N., R.N., C.S., F.N.P.
East Tennessee State University
Johnson City, TN

Carol Wysowski, B.S.N., R.N., C.R.N.I.
Wilkes-Barre General Hospital
Wilkes-Barre, PA

CHAPTER 1

Definitions and Historical Background

Instruments, tools, and machines have always been used in health care. In fact, whenever a new scientific discovery is made, whether it be in biology, chemistry, or physics, the health-care community tries to find ways to apply it to cures for disease or to wellness maintenance. For example, within weeks after their discovery in 1895, X rays were being used in bone imaging. Nuclear medicine was used before nuclear energy was practically applied in electrical power production or in the atomic bomb. This must have been true in the ancient world as well. Indeed, the motivation to find novel treatments for disease is very powerful.

There are two basic categories of medical instruments: those applied to applications of therapy and those used for diagnosis of disease.

Therapeutic instruments are the oldest. The basic process going on is the interaction between the machine and the human being, in this case for therapy. This interaction is basic to human life itself. The development of the thumb is certainly due in part to human manipulation of implements, first for food gathering and processing, then for shelter, then for transportation, health care, communication, and defense. The intimacy of the relationship between human beings and machines is illustrated by the fact that the thumb's motor nerves occupy a disproportionately large area of the brain. Among the machines that relate to human beings, none are more intimate than therapeutic medical machines, which are now implanted in the body and allow people who are dependent upon the machines for life to lead fully normal, active lives.

Therapeutic machines are physical structures that deliver physical substances to the body to treat disease. The physical substances include voltage, current, pressure, flow, force, ultrasound, radiation, and heat. The majority of the instruments discussed in this book will be in this category, and, therefore, the human–machine relationship will be emphasized.

1

Diagnostic instruments, the second category of medical devices, are those used to aid in the assessment of disease. They differ from therapeutic instruments in that they are designed to apply as little as possible of the physical substances just mentioned. Therefore, they are generally less invasive than therapeutic machines and pose fewer problems in the human–machine relationship.

HISTORICAL BACKGROUND

The number of medical instruments used in health care is so large that it is necessary to do a systematic study to understand the situation, and the complexities are so great that the quest for understanding can degenerate to just a desire to cope. The historical method is often used in health care, as when a patient's medical history is sought to diagnose illness and an understanding of that illness is sought through the study of its case history. Therefore, it is natural in the study of medical instrumentation to introduce it by a brief review of its history.

Therapeutic Instrumentation

Prior to the rise of science and the industrial revolution, most medical instruments were surgical implements for making incisions, cutting, grasping, probing, and prying. There is archeological evidence that even the Neanderthals did trephination, by boring a hole through the skull. New bone growth around the incision provided evidence that the subject survived. Surgical instruments used by the Romans and recovered as artifacts from the volcanic ashes include forceps for grasping, sharp spoons and probes, a trocar with a cannula for tapping fluids in cavities, a type of mirror called a speculum for examining the vagina and cervix, and a wound dilator.

People in this period used artificial dentures and glass magnifiers to aid in sight. As mechanical instruments were developed, they were inevitably modified and tried in health care. For example, Ambroise Pare (1510–1590) applied the principles of physics to properly arrange pulleys to set broken bones. He also made an early attempt to fashion artificial arms and hands for wounded soldiers using springs, gears, levers, and belts.

The instruments of obstetrics were improved by William Smelie (1697–1763), who developed new uses for the speculum and more invasive probes and forceps.

In the nineteenth century, surgical techniques were significantly advanced by the discovery of anesthetics like *ether* by William E. Clarke in 1842 and *chloroform* by John Snow in 1858. These are illustrated as one of the milestones in the development of modern medical instruments shown in Figure 1.1. The increased use of

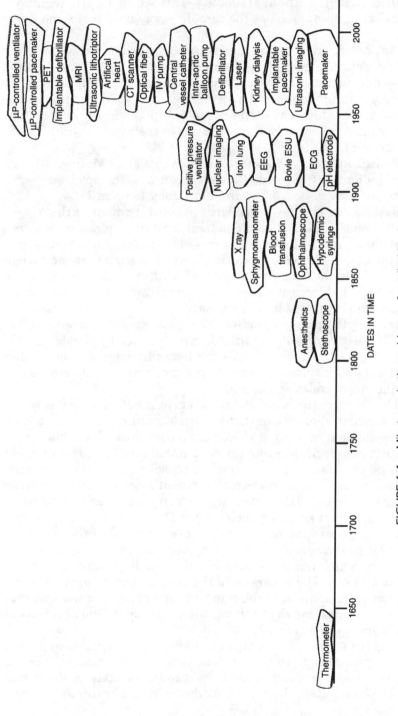

FIGURE 1.1 Milestones in the history of medical instrumentation.

surgery added to nosocomial infection spread by surgeons going from patient to patient without scrubbing. This led to aseptic technique and antiseptic spray, such as the carbolic spray used by Joseph Lister in 1870.

An adaptation of the suction pump to medical use resulted in the first *hypodermic syringe* by Alexander Wood in 1853. Techniques of hypodermic injection led to a portable patient-to-patient *blood transfusion apparatus* invented by James H. Aveling in 1863. Artificial pneumothorax, introduced by Carlo Fordanini in 1888, was achieved by injecting inert gas between the two layers of the pleura in order to collapse the rest of the lung.

Radiation therapy was begun three years after Marie Curie discovered radium in 1898, and ultraviolet light heat therapy began when Ernest Kromayer designed a *quartz ultraviolet lamp* in 1904.

Respiratory therapy began with the development of the *oxygen tent* by Leonard Hill in 1920. The treatment of respiratory paralysis with the *iron lung* followed in about 1928. This was an adaptation of the cylinder and the piston used in the syringe such that the patient was sealed from the neck down in the cylinder, and a piston was moved slightly back and forth at an appropriate breathing rate to move air in and out of the lung. This is called *negative pressure ventilation* because the piston applies pressure below atmospheric pressure, creating a suction. The *positive pressure ventilator* demonstrated by Guedel in 1934 used a compressor to drive air into the lung through the mouth. After the patient had inspired the breath, the machine would turn off and allow the lung to relax and exhale.

The therapeutic use of electrical current has been dramatically demonstrated in applications to the heart, beginning in 1956 with P. M. Zoll's application of short, high-current pulses through the chest wall to suppress heart fibrillation, uncoordinated heart palpitations that stop blood circulation. He also applied pulses of current through the chest wall to pace the heart at a higher rate in cases of bradycardia. The reliability of the *defibrillator* was significantly improved in 1962 when B. Lown demonstrated a device that put DC current pulses through the chest to defibrillate the heart. The development of the transistor in the 1950s led engineer Wilson Greatbatch to design an *implantable pacemaker*, which was demonstrated successfully by surgeon William Chardak in 1960. The generator of the current pacing pulse was implanted under the surface of the skin, and wire conductor was threaded through a catheter into the heart ventricle. The evolution of this pacemaker is shown in Figure 1.2.

This led to the process of central vessel catheterization (CVC), which may be considered the ultimate of machine invasion since the heart is the most sensitive and vital organ in the body. A slight mechanical, electrical, or chemical disturbance to the heart's surface can

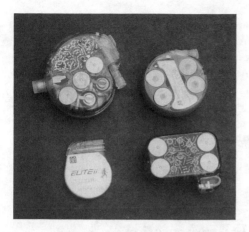

FIGURE 1.2 The size of the pacemaker has been reduced from the 1960s model in the upper left (going clockwise) to the modern pacemaker in the lower left corner. (Courtesy of Charles Verzi)

cause fibrillations that become fatal in minutes. The single lumen *central venous catheter* developed by Belding Scribner in the late 1960s made it possible to deliver nutrients and medications to the central veins with increased precision. The right atrial CVC was introduced by Robert Hickman in 1975. As a side effect, these catheters along with external pacemaker wires bypass the patient's natural defenses against microshocks (approximately one millionth of the current required to illuminate your living room). To overcome the increased back pressure in increasingly invasive intravenous (IV) therapy and to improve the precision for delivery of medications, *IV pumps* were developed in the 1970s.

Open-heart surgery was made possible by the introduction of *heart–lung bypass* apparatus introduced by H. Gibbon in 1953. This made possible artificial heart valve implantation and coronary artery bypass surgery. This development lead to development of the pneumatically driven *mechanical heart* first implanted into Barney Clark by W. C. DeVries and R. Jarvik in 1984.

Because of problems with the long-term biocompatibility of the complete artificial heart replacement, it is now considered a ventricular assist device, or bridge used until a heart transplant can be done. Ventricular assist devices began with the *intra-aortic balloon pump* (IABP) by A. Kantrowitz in 1967. This consists of a balloon implanted in the aorta that is timed to inflate when the aortic valve is closed, thus increasing blood flow.

An *artificial kidney* was introduced into clinical practice in 1960 by a group headed by B. H. Scribner that developed the technique of continuous hemodialysis. In this process, arterial blood is passed over a thin membrane, separating it from a cleansing solution that draws the blood waste products across the membrane by a diffusion process, thus replacing the kidney function.

Major developments in therapeutic instrumentation were made in the 1980s by the incorporation of the *microprocessor* into well-developed devices such as the pacemaker, IV pump, and ventilator. This has made it possible to program many different modes of operation, usually identified by acronyms, each of which has a different therapeutic effect. This has dramatically increased the complexity of these devices.

Almost all of the devices mentioned here, once introduced into health-care practice, have remained at least in some form and, therefore, accumulated in number. As a result, both the number of therapeutic devices and the complexity of the individual devices have greatly increased in recent years.

Diagnostic Instrumentation

Diagnostic instrumentation is designed to enhance the five senses to improve a health-care provider's ability to gather data for disease diagnosis. The speculum was used in Roman times to aid the physician in inspecting wounds and tissue. In 1625, Santorio Santorio used a *thermometer* to measure body temperature. This was a more objective means of assessing fever than touching the forehead with the hand. He also used a balance to monitor body weight. An early means of enhancing hearing was to use the hearing tube. In 1819, Rene T. H. Laennec is credited with inventing the *stethoscope*, which employed the same principle that operates in acoustic stethoscopes used today. Figure 1.3 shows a stethoscope in use.

As you can see, the diagnostic devices for primary care—the thermometer, scales, stethoscope, and speculum—have been used for hundreds of years in essentially the same form.

The first imaging of an internal organ not visible to the naked eye was probably done in 1851 by Hermann von Helmholtz when he invented the *ophthalmoscope* to inspect the retina of the eye. He used a mirror to direct light rays through the black pupil of the subject to illuminate the retina, thus making it visible to the observer. A much more dramatic enhancement of sight came in 1895 when Wilhelm Roentgen discovered *X rays* emitting from an electronic vacuum tube. He illustrated how these waves could produce images of bones underneath the skin with a picture of his wife's hand on film. Within weeks, X rays were being used to inspect bone injuries, thus illustrating how quickly esoteric advances in science have been put to use by health-care providers.

Early developments in electronics at the turn of the century led to the invention of the *electrocardiograph* (ECG) in 1903 by Willem Einthoven. This device measured the voltage produced between the limbs by the electrical activity of the heart. This is the first case of di-

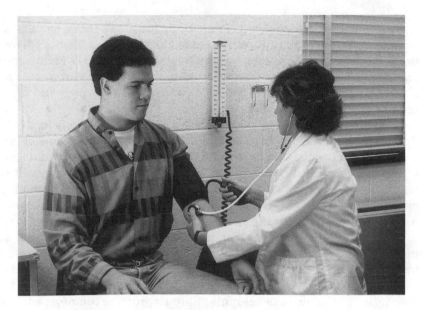

FIGURE 1.3   A stethoscope being used with a sphygmomanometer in a primary-care clinic

agnostic equipment that measures a physiological information parameter not directly perceivable by the human senses, at least to some degree. Further developments in electronic amplifiers led to the *electroencephalograph* (EEG) by Hans Berger in 1928. The EEG measured voltage potentials between anatomical sites on the skull and a neutral point, such as the ear, due to electrical activity of the brain. In both the case of the ECG and the EEG, the voltage levels were extremely small and represented major feats of measurement in their day.

Ultrasonic imaging devices have their roots in the sonar used in World War II to detect submarines and other obstructions underwater. Sound waves reflected from the boats could be measured to determine the size of the sound waves and the distance they were away. Likewise, the ultrasonic device tested for clinical applications by O. H. Houry and W. R. Bliss in 1957 detected heart valve activity and the position of anatomical structures like the midline of the brain.

Probably the most important recent advances in imaging have been computer based. The invention of the *microprocessor*, or computer on a chip, made it possible to replace, at a fraction of the cost, computers that occupied an entire room with desktop models of the same capability. That has made it possible for relatively small medical instruments to have their own dedicated computer. Such computers were used by Allan Cormack and Geoffrey Hounsfield in 1970 to create the computer tomography (CT) scanner for X-ray imaging. The CT scanner, which required instantaneous calculation of primary data to produce the image, became a commercial success and a widely applied clinical technique. The CT scanner measures the image of a cross section of the body, making it possible to inspect structures and organs hidden to a conventional X ray.

Likewise, the microprocessor and advances in magnets lead to the development of the *magnetic resonance imager* (MRI) in 1982. This device uses radio waves and a strong magnetic field to provide data from which the image can be calculated with its dedicated computer. It differs from the X ray in that bone is invisible to the MRI. Therefore, it gives better images of the brain and spinal cord. However, it cannot be used to inspect bone injuries as an X ray can.

Because the three imaging modalities—ultrasound, X ray, and magnetic resonance—are computer based, advances have been based on image processing and have been rapid in the 1980s. Research and development costs have contributed to the increasing cost of imaging for diagnosis. The goals of development are to produce the most accurate images with the least number of side effects to the patient and the costs kept under control.

Insights from History

The history of medical instrumentation shows that the number of medical instruments has progressively increased. This is clearly illustrated by the arrangement of the milestones in Figure 1.1. In fact, you can see an exponential growth in that figure. Furthermore, the complexity of the individual instruments has increased. Consequently, equipment management for health-care providers has become more complicated.

Over time the instrumentation has become more invasive as well. This has made the patient more vulnerable to side effects. For example, the increase in surgery due to the use of anesthetics in the nineteenth century led to more nosocomial infection. The response of the health-care community was to develop aseptic techniques during surgery. Likewise, the introduction of electronic devices into the operating room in the 1930s when flammable anesthetics were used led to fires and explosions. The health-care community responded with regulations and the establishment of the National Fire Protection Association (NFPA).

Equipment, such as ventilators, IV pumps, and CVCs, is more invasive and connects the patient to major hospital systems, such as the electrical power, the compressed air line, oxygen supplies, and computer networks. This has increased the safety problems. Microshock, for example, was unknown prior to the 1960s. But this equipment, which penetrates the skin and comes in close proximity to the heart, makes the patient vulnerable to a lethal response to currents only one millionth of the amount required to illuminate a small room.

The most invasive types of equipment are implanted devices, such as pacemakers, defibrillators, and central vessel catheters. They deliver therapeutic substances that are safe and effective only within a range. The doses and form of therapy is often controlled with microprocessors. This means that the complexity associated with the use of the equipment, and with keeping it safe and effective, has increased with time. Thus, the complexity of the equipment brings greater benefits to the patient but presents hazards as well. The defense of patient against this kind of hazard is best achieved through education. In other words, smarter machines require that people become smarter in the effective and safe use of them.

Machines and Information Processing

The purpose of machines has always been to extend human capabilities. The medical machine is almost always a physical structure that processes information from a living system that is used to produce a display of data for diagnosis or a substance for therapy. The *physical structure* consists of the nuts, bolts, resistors, capacitors, etc.; that is, the hardware. The *information* is contained in the variables that flow through the structure. The most common information variables in medical machines are pressure, fluid flow, voltage, and current. Definitions of the information variables are as follows:

Pressure—The force per unit area that tends to move matter, such as a fluid or a gas, from one point to another in a structure. Some units commonly used for pressure are pounds per square inch (psi), millimeters of mercury (mmHg), and Newtons per square meter (N/m^2).

Flow—The volume of fluid moved per unit time as a result of a pressure difference. Some units commonly used for flow are milliliters per second (ml/s) and cubic meters per second (m^3/s).

Voltage—The force that tends to move electric charges in an electrical circuit. This is sometimes called an electromotive force. Specifically, a volt is defined as the energy required to carry one coulomb of charge from ground to the point in the circuit where it is measured. A volt has units of joules per coulomb (J/C), where joules are the units of energy and coulombs are the units of electrical charge.

Current—An electrical current is defined as the number of coulombs of charge that flow per second (C/s) in an electrical circuit. The conventional direction of current flow is taken as positive in the direction that positive charges flow.

Power—Power is the rate at which energy, in units of joules, is delivered to tissue or to any other electrical resistance. It is equal to the voltage drop across the tissue times the current going through it. It has units of watts (W). The unit analysis is:

$$\frac{joules}{coulumb} \times \frac{coulumb}{second} = \frac{joule}{second} = watt$$

Energy—The electrical energy delivered to a tissue is equal to the power delivered times the time duration of delivery. Its units are joules. A dimensional analysis of the relationship of power to energy is:

$$\frac{joules}{seconds} \times seconds = joules$$

ELECTRICAL CIRCUIT COMPONENTS

The health-care provider attending the patient has primary responsibility for how the medical equipment is attached to the patient and how the patient is responding. The attendant needs to be confident that the attachments are safe; are as comfortable as possible; that they transfer accurate data to be used in patient testing, monitoring, and diagnosis; and that they deliver sufficient doses of substances used in therapy or surgery. To this end, it is beneficial to develop organizational principles so that the patient leads can be handled most effectively.

In the previous section, you learned that the information variables in the body include voltages and currents. The questions you should address now are: How are these quantities produced in the first place? How does the structure (in this case, the circuit) affect or process the values of these parameters? What are the elements of electrical circuit theory needed to help in the process of understanding how to deal with patient leads and medical equipment?

To answer the first question, start with the battery, an item with which all of you who use flashlights, Walkmans, or hand calculators are quite familiar. Although there are other ways to generate voltage, such as by electrical generators in the power station or by rubbing dissimilar materials together, the battery is featured because it creates voltage in a manner very similar to the way the body does as it produces a membrane voltage in a single cell.

The Battery

The electrical symbol for a battery is given in Figure 1.4. The two vertical lines represent metals that are immersed in an electrolyte. The cathode dissolves in the electrolyte, producing some free positive ions and an equal number of electrons. At the same time, a different type of metal in the anode combines free electrons with ions in the solution and deposits the metal on the anode. If a conduction path exists, as through the resistor, R, shown in Figure 1.4(b), the electrons will flow from the cathode through R to the anode. The process continues until all of the ions in the solution are exhausted. Then the battery is *discharged*. In rechargeable batteries, it is possible to reverse the process, so that the battery can be *recharged* to deliver current again. The *direction of conventional current flow* is defined as that of the positive ions in the electrolyte, which is opposite to the direction of the negatively charged electron flow in the wire and resistor.

Resistance

A common electrical resistor consists of a plastic tube filled with carbon and a conductor of electricity, as illustrated in Figure 1.5. The resistor is very much analogous to a blood vessel that passes blood through its resistance resulting from friction with the vessel walls. Your study of physiology revealed that blood vessels with smaller cross-sectional areas have higher resistance to blood flow. In other words, the resistance is inversely proportional to the cross-sectional area of the vessel. Furthermore, the longer the vessel, the higher the resistance; that is, the resistance is proportional to the length.

An similar situation exists in an electrical resistor. The formula for resistance is

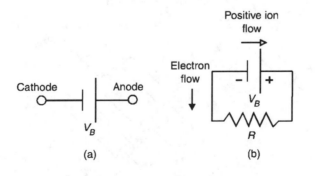

(a) (b)

FIGURE 1.4   Electrical symbol for a battery

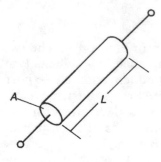

FIGURE 1.5   A resistor

$$R = \rho\frac{L}{A} \tag{1.1}$$

where L is the length of the resistor, A is the cross-sectional area, and ρ is the proportionality constant, called the resistivity.

When resistors are set in series, their length taken as a group increases (see Figure 1.6). So according to Equation (1.1), it is expected that the resistance would increase as well. In fact, the total resistance of resistors placed in series, R_T, is equal to the sum of the individual resistances. For example, for three resistors the formula is

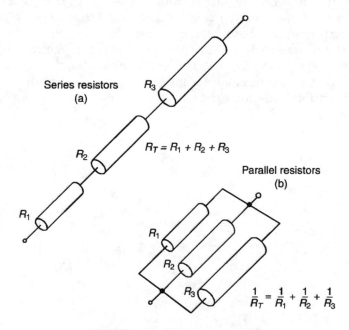

Series resistors (a)

$$R_T = R_1 + R_2 + R_3$$

Parallel resistors (b)

$$\frac{1}{R_T} = \frac{1}{R_1} + \frac{1}{R_2} + \frac{1}{R_3}$$

FIGURE 1.6   Resistor connections

$$R_T = R_1 + R_2 + R_3 \tag{1.2}$$

where R_1, R_2, and R_3 are the individual resistor values. This is also the case in the body for blood vessel resistance to blood flow. That is, the total resistance to the flow is equal to the sum of the resistance of the individual vessels connected in series, such as the artery, capillary, and vein in series. To be in series means that the current in each of the resistors is equal. Said another way, to be in series means that all of the current in one resistor goes into the resistor in series with it.

Another term for the element in Figure 1.5 is a *conductance*. A conductance, G, is defined as the inverse of the resistance. The formula is then

$$G = \frac{A}{\rho L} \tag{1.3}$$

When conductances are connected in parallel, it is clear that the area of the total conductance, G_T, is equal to the sum of the areas of the individual conductances. In other words, the reciprocal of the total resistance of resistors connected in parallel is equal to the sum of the reciprocals of the individual resistances. The formula for the total resistance, R_T, for three resistors connected in parallel as in Figure 1.6(b) is

$$\frac{1}{R_T} = \frac{1}{R_1} + \frac{1}{R_2} + \frac{1}{R_3} \tag{1.4}$$

where R_T is the total resistance and R_1, R_2, and R_3 are resistors in parallel, meaning they have the same voltage across them and are connected to the same nodes in the circuit.

To calculate the R_T on your hand calculator, it helps to rewrite Equation (1.4) in the form

$$R_T = \frac{1}{\dfrac{1}{R_1} + \dfrac{1}{R_2} + \dfrac{1}{R_3}} \tag{1.5}$$

Notice that the value of R_T is always going to be less than the value of any of the resistors connected in parallel.

ELECTRICAL CIRCUIT THEORY

The knowledge of a few simple electrical circuit theory concepts can reap tremendous benefits to the person who is responsible for the equipment leads attached to the patient. These ideas are powerful in the sense that they make orderly what would otherwise become confusing and entangled. You might think of them as housekeeping rules. Their use, therefore, improves the safety of the patient by giving protection against electrical shock and by building the confidence of the attendant who will feel personally certain of the patient's safety, the accuracy of the data, and the efficacy of the procedures and protocols.

Ohm's Law

The first idea is the duality of *cause and effect* in an electrical circuit. This idea holds in the fluidics concerning blood flow under pressure as well. If the pressure is higher at one point on a blood vessel than at another downstream, the pressure causes the blood to flow. But where is the pressure applied? It is applied at the heart muscle that is pushing the blood into the aorta. Downstream in the brachial artery in the arm, for example, the pressure at the heart will cause blood to flow. But at two separate points on the brachial, a difference of pressure can be measured. If the blood flow ceases, that pressure difference will go to zero. Thus, it is the flow that has caused the pressure difference.

By analogy, a voltage drop across a resistor causes a current to flow through it. But the converse is also true—the current in a resistor causes a voltage drop to appear across it. Figure 1.7 defines the relative direction of the current, I, through a resistor and the voltage drop, V, across it. A positive voltage in the direction plus (+) at the top to minus (–) at the bottom will cause a current of positive charges to flow in the direction of the arrow. Conversely, a current flowing in the direction of the arrow will cause a voltage drop to appear (+) on top of the resistor and (–) on the bottom. Furthermore, it was discovered by Georg Ohm (1787–1854) that the current flow through a resistor is proportional to the voltage drop across it. That is a statement of *Ohm's Law*. The formula is

$$V = IR \tag{1.6}$$

where the units on the voltage are called *volts* (symbolized with a V), the units on the current are called *amps* (symbolized with an I) and the units on the resistor, R, are called *ohms* (Ω).

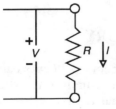

FIGURE 1.7   *Ohm's Law for a resistor*

EXAMPLE 1.1 In each case in Figure 1.8, calculate the current leaving the battery's positive terminal.

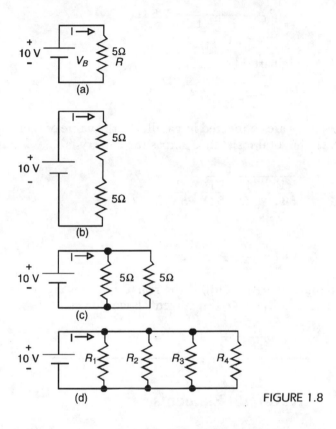

FIGURE 1.8

Solution a. In part (a) of the figure, the resistor is connected directly across the battery. Solving Ohm's Law, Equation (1.6), for the current yields

$$I = \frac{V_B}{R} = \frac{10 \text{ V}}{5 \text{ }\Omega} = 2 \text{ A}$$

b. In part (b), the two resistors are in series, so the total resistance is the sum

$$R_T = 5 \text{ }\Omega + 5 \text{ }\Omega = 10 \text{ }\Omega$$

From Ohm's Law, the current is then

$$I = \frac{V_B}{R_T} = \frac{10 \text{ V}}{10 \text{ }\Omega} = 1 \text{ A}$$

c. In part (c), the two resistors are in parallel. Thé total resistance using Equation (1.5) is

$$R_T = \frac{1}{\dfrac{1}{5\,\Omega} + \dfrac{1}{5\,\Omega}} = 2.5\ \Omega$$

Using this value of R_T as in part (b) gives

$$I = \frac{10\ \text{V}}{2.5\ \Omega} = 4\ \text{A}$$

d. In part (d), the resistors are connected in parallel. If the value of each of the resistors is 5 Ω, the total resistance across the battery is

$$R_T = \frac{1}{\dfrac{1}{5\,\Omega} + \dfrac{1}{5\,\Omega} + \dfrac{1}{5\,\Omega} + \dfrac{1}{5\,\Omega}} = 1.25\ \Omega$$

and

$$I = \frac{10\ \text{V}}{1.25\ \Omega} = 8\ \text{A}$$

In another example using part (d), if the resistor values are $R_1 = 2\ \Omega$, $R_2 = 3\ \Omega$, $R_3 = 5\ \Omega$, and $R_4 = 6\ \Omega$, the current, I, would be

$$I = \frac{10\ \text{V}}{0.833\ \Omega} = 12\ \text{A}$$

AC Circuit Elements

Current from a battery goes in only one direction as a function of time. Direct (DC) current, conventionally imagined to be a flow of positive charges, flows out of the positive terminal of the battery, through whatever resistance appears in the circuit, and into the negative terminal. The current available from the hospital wall-mounted receptacles is alternating (AC) current. It changes direction 60 times each second in step with the rotating electrical generator that produces it in the power station. The existence of AC currents and voltages gives rise to the concepts of capacitance and inductance.

Capacitance

A capacitor consists of any two pieces of metal separated by an insulator, such as air. As an electrical circuit element, it is usually thought of as two flat plates of metal separated by an insulator like paper or mica. Symbolically, it is represented by two parallel lines, as in Figure 1.9.

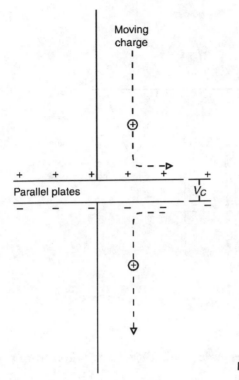

FIGURE 1.9   A capacitor

Imagine a positive charge moving onto the top plate. When it arrives, the force of its electrical field will repel a positive charge away from the lower plate, because like charges repel each other. In the direct current case, this process will continue until the voltage produced by the charge difference between the plates equals the applied voltage moving the charges onto the plate. At this point, the current will stop, and the capacitor is *charged*. In fact, when charged, the capacitor is storing energy, W_c, given by the formula

$$W_C = \frac{1}{2} C V_C^2 \quad \text{joules} \qquad (1.7)$$

where C is the value of the capacitor in farad (F) units, V_c is the voltage in volts, and energy W_c is in units called joules.

In the alternating current case, the process illustrated in Figure 1.10 repeats in cycles following the changes in polarity of the applied voltage with time. Above (a) in Figure 1.10, the charges are entering the top plate and leaving the bottom plate. Applied voltage is positive. Above (b) in Figure 1.10, the charges are entering the bottom plate and leaving the top plate. The V_c is negative. Above (c) in Figure 1.10, the

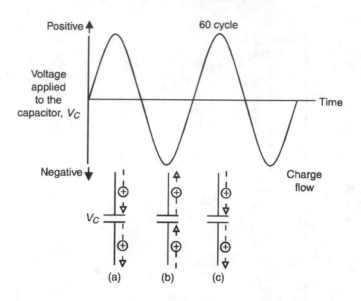

FIGURE 1.10   AC current in a capacitor

cycle repeats, usually at 60 cycles per second for voltage taken from a wall power receptacle.

This figure illustrates how AC current flows through a capacitor, while the previous figure illustrates how current is stopped by the capacitor once it is charged. The mechanism for the conduction of AC current through the capacitor is the *changing* electrical field associated with the charge that collects on the plates. In other words, it is only when the voltage is changing as a function of time that current flows through a capacitor.

Just as a capacitance exists between two parallel metal plates, it also exists between any two conductors separated by an insulator. For example, a capacitance exists between a person in a room and the power lines that feed the wall-mounted receptacles. A person has electrolytes in the interstitial fluid under the skin, which is one conductor. The metal of the power cables is the other conductor. Thus, separated by air, the capacitance is formed. The hospital, being a high-tech building, has many power lines. Therefore, the capacitance between the patients and the power circuits is appreciable, in the order of several picofarads (10^{-12} farads). In fact, 60-cycle currents are induced in people both in the hospital and in any other buildings with electrical power. The physiological effects of such currents, minute as they are, are under study. There is concern that they could cause cancer, especially in high-exposure cases, such as in power line repair people. These studies are inconclusive at the present time.

Inductance

Michael Faraday (1791–1867) made two basic observations regarding electrical current flow. First, he showed that a current in a wire causes a magnetic field in the medium surrounding it. Second, he discovered that a *change* in the magnetic field strength passing through a wire connected from one end to the other end of a resistor will cause a current in that wire and resistor. Such a change may be induced by an AC current. This process is called induction, as measured by the *inductance* associated with AC currents.

One widely used application of inductance is in transformer action, as illustrated in Figure 1.11. An AC transformer consists of a coil of wire wound on a core on which another coil is also wound. Current, I_{IN}, passing through the primary coil on the left of the core induces a magnetic field flux, φ, in the core, usually made of iron. If I_{IN} is an AC current, it will induce an alternating magnetic flux into the core. The changing magnetic field, cutting the secondary coil on the right, will induce an AC current, I_{OUT}, in the coil that flows through the resistor.

Notice there is no transfer of conduction charges from the primary circuit to the secondary circuit. This is an example of force operating at a distance, and such forces are always a little mysterious. Another example of force that operates at a distance is the force of gravity. In fact, radio waves propagating through space is another case of currents being induced from one conductor into another, the conductors being the two antennas involved.

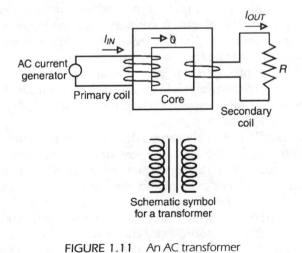

FIGURE 1.11   An AC transformer

AC Power Lines

Hospital AC power lines, accessible through a wall-mounted receptacle into which one plugs most portable medical devices, usually receive their electrical current from the local power company. The current from the outside power lines is tapped into a transformer, as illustrated in Figure 1.12.

The transformer reduces the voltage of the outside power lines to either 110 V AC or 220 V AC at the power mains and wall receptacle. Virtually all portable AC medical equipment runs off 110 V AC. High-power equipment will sometimes use 220 V AC. The plugs on the two different types of equipment are different, so one cannot plug it into the wrong receptacle. A schematic for the 110 V AC 60-cycle, three-wire power line (the power main) that runs behind the hospital walls is shown in Figure 1.12. The secondary coil of the transformer is connected to the hot (H) and neutral (N) wires. The N wire is connected to a separate ground (G) wire near the power service entrance. The G wire is in turn connected to a pipe driven into the earth. The earth, or ground, is moist, contains electrolytes, and is a conductor of electricity. It is used universally as a reference for power circuits.

The wall receptacle is connected to the hospital power line. The receptacle is wired in accordance with a power cord color code as follows:

Hot wire—black

Neutral wire—white

Ground wire—green

The connections to the receptacle are as follows: The H wire is connected to the short rectangular receptor on your upper right as you face the receptacle. The N wire is connected to the longer rectangular receptor on the upper left. The G wire is connected to the rounded receptor on the middle lower part of the receptacle.

The plug has prongs of the proper shape and orientation so that the plug will fit into the receptacle in only one orientation. This feature prevents accidental miswiring of the equipment attached to the hospital AC power receptacle.

You are familiar with electronic devices such as radios, video cassette recorders, kitchen appliances, blow-dryers, and bath accessories. The issues that pertain to the equipment used in daily life also apply to medical instruments. For example, in the home, the hazards of equipment used in the living room are different from those used in the bathroom, where a person is much more exposed and vulnerable. In the hospital, these issues become even more serious because of the increased vulnerability of the patient and the greater need for accuracy.

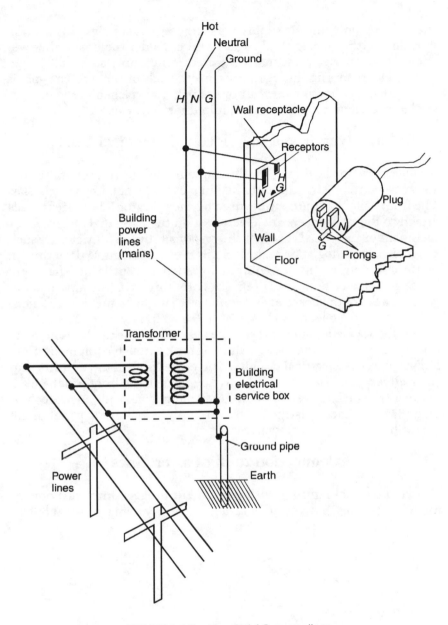

FIGURE 1.12   Hospital AC power lines

THE MEDICAL INSTRUMENT AS A UNIT

The medical instrument as it is used at the patient's bedside is encased in a box. The attendant should have a clear idea of how the instrument is plugged into such hospital systems as the electrical power supply, the water supply, the air supply, and the oxygen supply. This section will deal with the electrical supply and consider the hospital power supply as discussed previously, the electronic unit itself, and the patient attachments (in this case, the patient leads or tubing). The goal is to ensure the safety and comfort of the patient attached to the unit, as well as the accuracy of the data acquired for diagnosis.

An Overview of the Electronic Medical Unit

An electronic medical unit, as illustrated in Figure 1.13, generally consists of electronic circuits contained in a case surrounding the chassis. The front panel has the controls used by the operator. The patient leads attach to the transducers and electrodes on the patient. The proper attachment of these leads is often the responsibility of a specialist, such as an electrocardiography technician, but often the nurse does this. In fact, increasingly complex equipment, such as ventilators that were formerly used only in the intensive care unit (ICU), is now used in general areas of the hospital and sometimes in the home, where a nonspecialist nurse becomes responsible for it. In any case, it is often a nurse who specializes in the task. These attachments can become complicated and require that one be able to think through equipment problems and follow electrical circuits. The power plug of the unit fits into the wall receptacle for electrical current. Also on the front panel are adjustments, which are usually made by a biomedical equipment technician (BMET). The adjustments are often placed behind a panel or are accessible only with a screwdriver.

Connection to the Power Lines

You are no doubt familiar with equipment plugged into wall power-main receptacles, but you may seldom think systematically about it.

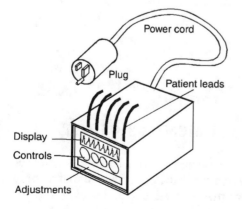

FIGURE 1.13   A medical equipment unit

Figure 1.14 shows how the electronic chassis is connected to the hospital power source. In part (a), a three-wire connection is shown. The *H* wire and the *N* wire are connected to the electronic circuit boards, and the *G* wire is connected to both the circuit boards and the chassis, grounding them both. The *H* wire and the *N* wire provide the high currents necessary to run the equipment. The *G* lead is there for safety to reduce voltage elevation of the chassis, leakage, and the danger of electrical shocks to personnel. It can happen that in operating the equipment one makes contact with a metal conductor, such as a switch. Even a plastic dial might have a metal screw in it which would make an electrical connection, all of which would be grounded as long as the *G* wire remains intact.

Another safe connection is the double-insulated arrangement shown in part (b) of Figure 1.14. Here the *H* wire and the *N* wire go to the electronic circuit boards. These boards are grounded by the *N* wire, which is connected to ground at the electrical service box, as explained in the previous section. To be certain that no electricity is conducted to the case, even if it is metal, the inside is coated with a nonconductor, such as plastic. In this case, all dials and switches on the front panel would also be nonconductors or somehow insulated.

Another two-wire connection puts the *H* wire and the *N* wire on the electronics circuit board, which is insulated from the case and controls. This is shown in part (c) of Figure 1.14. However, the insu-

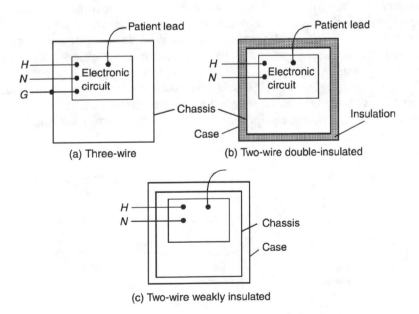

FIGURE 1.14   Types of power connections

lation can easily become fouled by oil, grime, or body fluids and cannot be trusted in the hospital situation. Some of this equipment may have large metal surfaces, such as a metal chassis, grounded through the N wire. To prevent a reversal of the H wire and the N wire, the prongs to the plug are shaped as shown in Figure 1.15 (a). Such a reversal would put 110 volts on the chassis and increase the risk of a high-voltage shock. Unfortunately, much commercial equipment uses a plug like the one shown in Figure 1.15(b), where the prongs are the same size and reversals of the H wire and the N wire occur half the time. The three-prong plug in part (c) of the figure accommodates the ground wire.

Chassis Voltage Elevation

Small voltage elevations on the chassis of much commercially available electronics equipment are tolerable because the equipment does not normally contact the human body. Medical equipment, however, is often grounded directly to the patient's body, and the chassis and voltage elevations become hazardous. Figure 1.16(a) illustrates how voltage elevations can occur between different two-wire equipment attached to the same hospital power line. The voltage elevation occurs because the high current needed to operate the equipment flows in the H wire and out the N wire. This large current causes a voltage to develop between the equipment and the ground to which the N wire is connected. Therefore, the ground reference of the equipment becomes elevated in voltage from that of other objects in the room connected to the earth, such as water pipes and heating radiators. So, if you put a voltmeter between the water pipe and a two-wire equipment chassis, you will probably measure nearly one volt. Furthermore, different equipment on the same hospital power line will carry different currents and acquire different voltage levels. Thus, you would also measure a voltage difference between various equipment chassis in the room. Example 1.2 illustrates this.

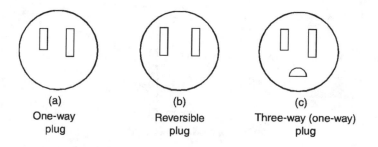

(a)
One-way
plug

(b)
Reversible
plug

(c)
Three-way (one-way)
plug

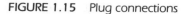

FIGURE 1.15   Plug connections

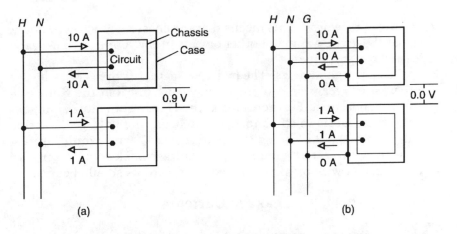

FIGURE 1.16   Voltage problem and cure

EXAMPLE 1.2   In Figure 1.16(a), the upper equipment has 10 A going in the H lead and out the N wire, which has 0.1 Ω resistance from the equipment to the hospital power line. Therefore, because of Ohm's Law, the voltage drop is

$$0.1 \, \Omega \times 10 \, A = 1 \, V$$

But the lower equipment draws only 1 A so its voltage drop to the hospital power line is

$$0.1 \, \Omega \times 1 \, A = 0.1 \, V$$

Therefore, the voltage between the chassis of the two pieces of equipment is

$$1 \, V - 0.1 \, V = 0.9 \, V$$

When the physiological effect of electricity on the body is discussed in the next section, you will see that in medical practice, even such a low voltage difference can be dangerous. To eliminate these voltage elevations, a three-wire power cord is used for the equipment, as illustrated in Figure 1.16(b). Here, the high currents needed to run the equipment enter the H lead and exit the N lead, but no current goes through the G lead. The G lead in both cases is connected to the chassis. Therefore, the voltage elevation between the two pieces of equipment is zero. Furthermore, since under normal circumstances, the G wire in the hospital power line does not carry current, it will not develop a voltage drop. This means that the chassis voltage will not be elevated above the ground of other objects in the room, such as water pipes and radiator pipes.

That's the good news. The bad news is that if the *G* wire breaks due to wear and tear, the equipment may work fine, but the voltage elevations may return. Furthermore, if the *H* lead somehow short-circuits to the chassis in an abnormal situation, the voltage elevation could go to 110 V on the chassis. An intact *G* wire would protect against such a hazard by reducing the voltage back to near zero. To guard against *G* wire breakage, periodic inspections should be made.

Leakage Currents

Leakage currents are currents that flow out of the power cables into the ground. Most of the leakage is due to the fact that the wires are made of metal and are separated from the metal of the chassis, from other wires, and from the ground itself. These two metal surfaces, separated by an insulator, make up a capacitance. The AC power currents flow through this capacitance as was explained by Figure 1.10. Figure 1.17 illustrates the various paths for leakage current due to stray capacitance in medical equipment. Leakage can pass from the chassis wiring to the ground and from the *H* wire to the patient lead. In Figure 1.17, a patient would get leakage current from the patient lead when touching ground. Or the leakage could flow through an attendant who touches the equipment and the patient at the same time. Leakage current due to stray capacitance can never be totally eliminated in equipment powered by 60-cycle power lines, just as you can never get rid of all of the friction in a machine. As long as metal is involved, the capacitance will be there. However, it can be reduced to

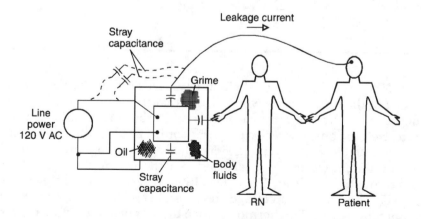

FIGURE 1.17   Leakage current paths

safe levels, as explained in the following section. There is also some leakage current due to transformer action between adjacent conductors carrying AC currents. The capacitance however, is usually the larger effect.

The other largest contributor of leakage current is resistance. Normally, the insulation on the wires passes some minute current. However, larger amounts of current can be carried by dirt, grime, and body fluids that may get into the equipment. Equipment ventilator fans may pull dust and oil from the air into the equipment. These deposits build up conduction paths that create leakage currents in all of the places just mentioned. As the equipment ages, it gets dirtier, the insulation gets brittle, and leakage currents develop. To protect against this, periodic measurement of the leakage currents should be done biannually or annually. Of course, leakage current due to dirt can be eliminated by cleaning.

ELECTRICAL SHOCK

An *electrical shock* is any unwanted physiological response to an electrical current applied to the body. The physiological responses of an electrical current in the body begin at the cellular level. A current passing in the vicinity of a single cell will depolarize it if it is above threshold. Here is how this happens: The cell at rest is *polarized*, which means it exhibits a resting membrane potential of approximately 90 mV, polarized negative on the inside with respect to the outside. The cell stimulated by a current creates an *action potential*. An action potential is a transient during which the membrane potential goes to approximately 10 mV of the opposite polarity. During this time, the cell is said to be *depolarized*. After the transient in the order of 10 to 300 ms, the cell returns to the polarized rest state. In a muscle cell, this process will cause a contraction of the muscle. If this contraction is unwanted, it would be called an electrical shock.

If the current applied to the body is large enough, it can cause the cell to get hot and ultimately to vaporize. This form of an electrical shock would be manifested as tissue injury. In summary, a shock appears as unwanted tissue stimulation, unwanted muscle contraction, or tissue injury.

The danger of an electrical shock increases as the current level increases. Shock is measured in terms of current rather than voltage because the physiological responses of the body are consistantly related to current intensity. Shocks of current confined to the limbs may cause injury but are less dangerous than shocks to the vital regions of the heart and the respiratory centers. Currents passing through the heart or brain stem can cause death.

Currents Applied to the Surface of the Body

Currents will pass through the vital organs of circulation and respiration if one side of the source is applied to one limb and the other side is applied to another limb. Such currents would pass through the thorax and therefore affect the heart or respiratory muscles. Another path through the vital organs is from any limb to the neck or head. Another path through vital organs is from the head to the neck or below. However, currents traveling from the biceps brachii to a hand or between two abdominal sites would not cause life-threatening effects of respiratory paralysis or heart failure, provided they were not so large as to diffuse into the vital regions.

The path of the current from arm to arm is illustrated in Figure 1.18. Estimates of the effects of passing this current from a 60-cycle power bus between the two arms of a 150-pound person for at least 1 to 3 seconds are given as follows (see Olsen):

> *1–5 mA*—Just above the threshold level of feeling. These currents are not considered hazardous.

> *5–8 mA*—A range in which the physiological effect is pain. Tissue damage usually occurs, resulting in redness after prolonged application. Currents above 5 mA are considered dangerous.

> *8–20 mA*—The range of involuntary muscle contraction. A level of 8 mA is the threshold of *let-go* current, which is the current level above which a person cannot let go of the current source if it is applied to the hands because the muscles are involuntary contracted by the current.

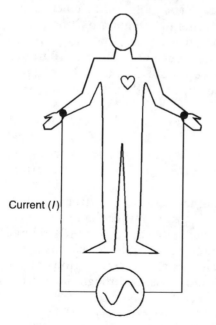

Current (*I*)

FIGURE 1.18   Current passed from arm to arm

20 mA and above—Respiratory paralysis and a cessation of breathing are caused. This level of current in the arms causes sufficient current density at the respiratory centers in the brain stem and at the respiratory muscles to paralyze them. Death will occur in several minutes if the current is not removed. Although spontaneous recovery can occur after the source of shock is removed, artificial respiration is recommended for resuscitation.

80 mA to 1 A—Fibrillation of the heart is caused. This level of current in the arms produces sufficient current densities in the heart to disrupt the normal depolarization sequence. Several ectopic centers take over the function of the SA node as the pacemaker of the heart. The contraction of various muscles in the heart becomes uncoordinated, causing the heart to lose its effectiveness as a pump for blood. This condition is fatal in minutes. Furthermore, a fibrillating heart will not recover spontaneously when the source of shock is removed.

1 A to 10 A—Sustained myocardial contraction is caused. This means that the heart is not beating while the current is applied. After the source of shock is removed, the heart may spontaneously recover its beat. However, long durations of current would cause surface tissue burns. Electronic defibrillators for resuscitating the heart work on this principle but have carefully controlled currents, as will be discussed in Chapter 6.

In summary, it is clear that currents above 5 mA applied to the surface of the body should be considered hazardous. Currents above 20 mA that pass through a vital organ will cause electrocution if they are not removed in time. The physiological effects of currents in excess of 5 mA are called *macroshocks,* because they are large currents applied to the surface of the body. These effects occur for current durations greater than 1 second. If the duration of the current is reduced, the effects will likewise reduce. For example, the fibrillation threshold increases ten times if the current duration is reduced to 0.1 second. This fact is used to design circuit interrupters to prevent injuries due to shock, as will be discussed in the next chapter.

Microshock and Macroshock*

A much subtler electrical shock situation than macroshock is *microshock*. It is sometimes more dangerous because it is difficult to detect. The two situations differ as indicated by the following definitions:

*This section is reprinted with permission of Merrill, an imprint of Macmillan Publishing Company, from *Principles of Biomedical Instrumentation and Measurements* by Richard Aston, copyright 1990 by Macmillan Publishing Company, pp. 55–56.

Macroshock—A physiological response to a current applied to the surface of the intact skin of the *body* that produces unwanted or unnecessary stimulation, muscle contractions, or tissue injury.

Microshock—A physiological response to a current applied to the surface or in the close vicinity of the *heart* that produces unwanted stimulation, muscle contractions, or tissue injury.

Microshock is most often caused when currents in excess of 10 μA flow through an insulated catheter to the heart, as illustrated in Figure 1.19. The catheter may be an insulated, conductive-fluid-filled tube or a solid-wire pacemaker cable, as illustrated in Figure 1.19(a). The microshock results because the current density at the heart can become high when the catheter is touching the heart. To produce macroshock, a much larger current is required because the current distributes itself throughout the body, as shown in Figure 1.19(b). Obviously, the current density at the heart is much lower in this case, and more current is required to cause a shock. This accounts for the thousand-to-one ratio of macroshock to microshock current levels.

Shocks from Equipment

Normally, equipment is designed not to shock a patient. However, certain failures, called *faults*, can occur and give a patient a macroshock. For example, if the *H* wire accidently contacts a patient lead, the patient would obviously receive a macroshock. Another example of macroshock would be when a patient is attached to two pieces of equipment. Suppose one piece of equipment (Equip. #1 in Figure 1.20) is in very bad condition and the *H* wire is shorted to the

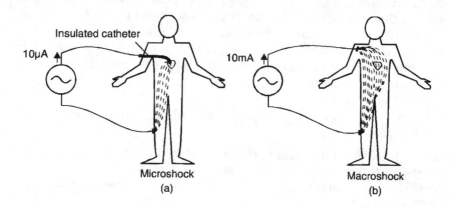

FIGURE 1.19   *The current density accompanying microshock versus that accompanying macroshock*

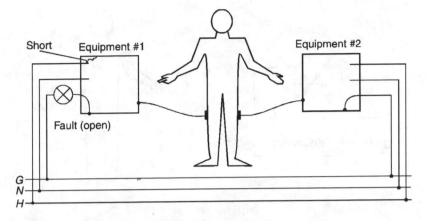

FIGURE 1.20   An example of macroshock

chassis, while the G lead that is connected to the chassis is open. Another device (Equip. #2 in Figure 1.20) is normal and connected to the patient. Both pieces of equipment are plugged into the wall receptacles. The macroshock current path is from the H lead of Equip. #1 to its chassis to the patient then into the ground lead of Equip. #2 and back to ground through its G wire. This macroshock would not occur if the G wire of Equip. #1 was intact. In that case, the H wire would be shorted to the ground, and the circuit breaker would be tripped. This illustrates how important the G wire is as a protection against macroshock.

Microshock can occur in equipment when dirt and grime build up between the H wire and the chassis, or between the H wire and the patient lead. Examples 1.3 and 1.4 illustrate this.

EXAMPLE 1.3   A patient is connected to a pressure monitor by way of a catheter. Dirt and grime make a resistance path from the catheter to the H wire of 500,000 Ω. The H wire is plugged into a 110 V power bus. In Figure 1.21, the series circuit carrying the leakage current to the patient has resistances as follows:

H wire to patient lead	500,000 Ω
Catheter	5,000 Ω
Viscera resistance	200 Ω
Return electrode resistance	10,000 Ω
Total	515,200 Ω

The driving voltage across this 515.2 kilohms (k Ω) resistance is the 110 V on the H wire. Thus, by Ohm's Law, there is a leakage current, I_L, of

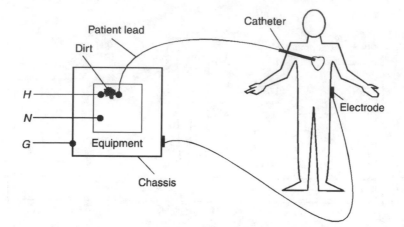

FIGURE 1.21

$$I_L = \frac{110 \text{ V}}{515,200 \ \Omega} = 0.000213 \text{ A} = 213 \ \mu\text{A}$$

This example illustrates how 213 μA of leakage current could pass into the heart of a patient. This exceeds the 10 μA safe limit and could cause a heart fibrillation. This is a case where with all of the wires intact, the equipment has developed an excessive leakage current due to dirt buildup.

Example 1.4 shows how dirt could cause excessive leakage current when two pieces of equipment are attached to the same patient.

EXAMPLE 1.4   In this case, two pieces of equipment are attached to the patient, as shown in Figure 1.22. In Equip. #1 dirt has built up a path from the H wire to the chassis of 200 kΩ. Also, this equipment has a faulty G wire that is open in the power cord. The patient is grounded to another piece of equipment. An RN is threading a catheter into the patient's heart and, at the same time, is touching the chassis of Equip. #1. In Figure 1.22, a circuit carries a leakage current to the patient through the following resistances:

H lead to chassis	200	kΩ
RN skin resistance (right hand)	20	kΩ
RN skin resistance (left hand)	20	kΩ
Catheter resistance	5	kΩ

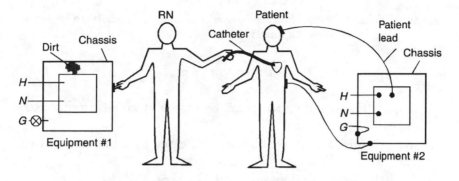

FIGURE 1.22   Attendant-mediated microshock

Patient viscera resistance	0.2 kΩ
Patient return electrode	10 kΩ
Total	255.2 kΩ

The driving voltage across this 255.2 kΩ of resistance is 110 V. Therefore, by Ohm's Law, there is a leakage current of

$$I_L = \frac{110 \text{ V}}{255.2 \text{ k}\Omega} = 0.000431 \text{ A} = 431 \text{ μA}$$

The leakage current of 431 μA exceeds the safe limit of 10 μA. Currents of this level applied directly to the heart could cause a fibrillation. In this case, if the G wire were not broken, this leakage current would not get to the patient.

REFERENCES

Bettmann, Otto. *A Pictorial History of Medicine: A Brief Non-Technical Survey of Healing Arts From Aesculapires to Ehrlich.* Springfield, Ill.: Thomas, 1956.

Bronzino, J. D. *Biomedical Engineering and Instrumentation.* Boston: Prindle, Weber & Schmidt, 1986.

Carr, J. J., and John Brown. *Introduction to Biomedical Equipment Technology.* New York: John Wiley & Sons, 1981.

Olsen, W. H. "Electrical Safety," Chapter 14 in *Medical Instrumentation: Application and Design.* Edited by J. G. Webster. Boston: Houghton-Mifflin Company, 1993.

Reiser, Stanley Joel. *Medicine and the Reign of Technology.* Cambridge, UK: Cambridge University Press, 1978.

Singer, Charles. *A Short History of Medicine.* New York: Oxford University Press, 1962.

Venzmer, Gerhard. *Five Thousand Years of Medicine*. Translated by Marion Koenig. New York: Taplinger, 1972.

EXERCISES

1. What information variables are processed by an electronic instrument?
2. What information variables are processed by a hydraulic instrument?
3. Identify the three components of a battery.
4. Define the direction of conventional current flow.
5. Increasing what dimension of a carbon-filled resistor gives it a smaller value?
6. Increasing what dimension of a carbon-filled resistor gives it a larger value?
7. Define a conductance in terms of a resistor.
8. State Ohm's Law.
9. The voltage drop across a 15-Ω resistor is 30 V. What is the current through it?
10. The current through a 15 ohm resistor is 0.5 A. What is the corresponding voltage drop?
11. Two resistors are connected in series. One of them is 10 Ω and the total resistance is 25 Ω. What is the value of the other resistance?
12. Three 10-Ω resistors are connected in parallel. What is the value of the total resistance?
13. Three resistors are connected in parallel. They have values 10 Ω, 5 Ω, and 15 Ω. What is the value of the total resistance?
14. Three resistors are connected in parallel. The values of two of them are 20 Ω and 15 Ω. The total resistance of the three resistors is 5 Ω. What is the value of the other resistor?
15. In each case in Figure 1.23, find the value of current I as indicated by the open arrow.

    (a) $I =$ (b) $I =$
    (c) $I =$ (d) $I =$
    (e) $I =$

16. In each case in Figure 1.24, find the value of the voltage across the element as indicated by V.

    (a) $V =$ (b) $V =$
    (c) $V_1 =$ (d) $V_2 =$
    (e) $V =$

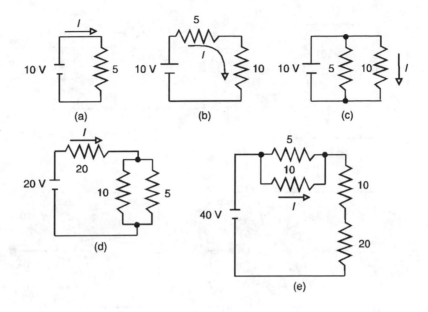

FIGURE 1.23

17. Fill in the blanks of the voltage division rule as follows: The voltage drop across one of several resistors in series equals the resistance the _____ is dropped across divided by the total ____ times the input voltage dropped across the total _____. (Refer to the Appendix).

18. Fill in the blanks about the current division rule as follows: The current through one of two resistors in parallel equals the value of the _____ opposite the one conducting the current in question divided by sum of the two _____ times the _____ entering the node connecting the two resistors. (Refer to the Appendix).

19. Dirt and grime have gotten into the casing of a hospital-bed motor, making a 350 kΩ connection between the *H* wire and the bed's metal frames. An attendant has one hand on the bed's metal frame and the other on a bare-wire pacemaker lead to the patient's heart. The patient is connected to the ground lead of an ECG monitor. The bed is powered by 110 V AC. The resistances are as follows:

H lead to bed metal	350	kΩ
RN skin resistance (each hand)	30	kΩ
Pacemaker lead resistance	5	kΩ
Viscera resistance	0.3	Ω
Patient skin resistance		
to the monitor ground lead	10	kΩ

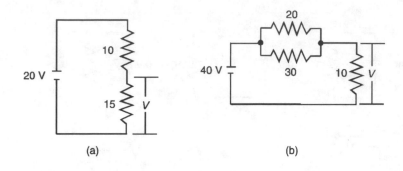

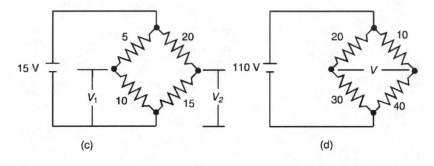

FIGURE 1.24

What leakage current flows into the patient's heart from this effect? What would be the probable physiological response of the patient to that leakage current?

20. Body fluids have gotten into a pressure monitor connected to a patient, creating a 500 kΩ resistance between the H lead and the patient lead, which is connected to a catheter touching the patient's heart. The listing of the resistances from the 110 V H lead to ground is as follows:

H lead to patient lead	500 kΩ
Catheter resistance	5 kΩ
Viscera resistance	10 kΩ
Monitor ground electrode	15 kΩ

What leakage current flows into the patient's heart from this effect? What would be the probable physiological response of the patient to that leakage current?

CHAPTER 2

Hospital Equipment Safety

The hospital is a place where highly educated and trained people are dedicated to providing medical and surgical treatment to patients who cannot be treated as effectively in the home. The success of the treatment is measured by extended life expectancy and freedom from disease and infirmity. The staff is committed to providing treatment that improves or maintains health, in accordance with the oath of Hippocrates, without intending any harm to the patient. The patient, however, is often in a vulnerable position in the hospital because treatment or surgery may require that natural defenses against injury, poisoning, infection, or electrical shock be bypassed. When the skin is broken, for example, one is more vulnerable to infection and electrical shock. Under anesthesia, the patient loses consciousness and pain awareness, and needs other protection against all hazards. To defend the patient against these hazards places a burden on the health-care professional.

In the second half of the twentieth century, the number and complexity of machines used in health care have increased dramatically. In particular, the microprocessor on a chip of silicon only one or two square inches in area has increased the complexity available by 10,000 times, as measured by the parts density of electronic equipment over mechanical devices. This has made the problem of controlling the adverse side effects and complications of medical equipment more difficult. For example, microshock was unknown and not a problem before the 1960s when central venous catheterization was introduced. Furthermore, a change in the dial settings of complex critical-care equipment, such as external pacemakers and ventilators, can introduce dangerous complications. To understand these situations requires systematic study of both the physiology of the patient and the characteristics of the machine involved.

The purpose of this chapter is to determine how safety can be maintained when the patient is vulnerable to electrical shock, injury, toxic materials, and fire. These hazards will be described, as will be the procedures and mechanisms.

ELECTRICAL SHOCK SITUATIONS

In Chapter 1, electrical shock was defined in terms of current delivered to the body. A macroshock usually results from a current greater than 5 mA delivered to the surface of the body. A microshock may result from a current greater than 10 µA delivered to the surface of the heart. These currents are considered dangerous.

Tissue Resistance

Skin resistance is measured in ohms per square centimeter of area (ohm/cm^2). When measured with a 1-cm^2 electrode, its value varies from 10 kΩ to several hundred kΩ, depending upon the condition of the skin; that is, whether there is perspiration, a callus, or tender skin. A disposable pre-gelled stainless steel electrode has an electrode-to-skin resistance of approximately 97 kΩ/cm^2, and a self-adhesive gum electrode has an impedance of about 144 kΩ/cm^2 (see Carim). Dry skin typically measures 100 kΩ/cm^2; but when it is vigorously rubbed with salty gel it drops to 10 kΩ/cm^2, at a frequency of 60 cycles per second. The hierarchy of tissue resistances from highest to lowest is as follows:

Skin

Fat

Lung

Muscle

Blood

Taken as a whole, the resistance of the viscera underneath the skin is in the order of 200 ohms. Salty gel is effective in reducing skin resistance, and vigorous rubbing makes it even more conductive.

From these data you can calculate what the resistance of an electrode ought to be, depending upon its area. According to Equation (2.1), the resistance is inversely proportional to the area. Therefore, doubling the area of the electrode reduces its resistance by half. In general, use the following formula to estimate electrode resistance, R_E:

$$R_E = \frac{\text{Resistance for 1 square centimeter}}{\text{Electrode area in square centimeters}} \qquad (2.1)$$

Using the data given above, this formula can be used to estimate the resistance of a gelled ECG electrode or a defibrillator paddle.

EXAMPLE 2.1 A conductive-gelled ECG electrode has an area of 10 cm², and a gelled defibrillator paddle has an area of 80 cm². If, under pressure, the skin-electrode resistance is 10.8 kΩ/cm², estimate the resistance of these electrodes when placed on the body, as illustrated in Figure 2.1.

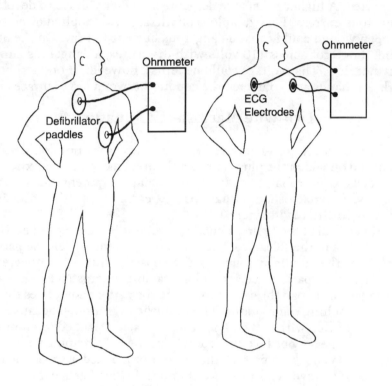

FIGURE 2.1   Defibrillator paddles compared to ECG electrodes

Solution   Using Equation (2.1), for the ECG electrode

$$R_E = \frac{10.8 \text{ kohms}}{10} = 1{,}080 \text{ ohms}$$

and for the defibrillator paddles

$$R_E = \frac{10.8 \text{ kohms}}{80} = 135 \text{ ohms}$$

Example 2.1 shows that a defibrillator paddle, being eight times larger than an ECG electrode, presents one-eighth the resistance.

Dangerous Voltage Levels

What is considered to be a dangerous voltage applied to the surface of the body depends upon the resistance. It is the current that causes the shock response. According to Ohm's Law, the voltage required to drive the dangerous current through the body depends on the resistance encountered. A higher resistance demands a higher voltage to develop a dangerous current. For example, as little as 1 volt applied directly to an open wound could cause a dangerous current to flow. On the other hand, if one got across 110 volts with dry hands, a dangerous current may not flow. That voltage could be lethal, however, if one grabbed it with wet hands and contacted the conductor over a large surface area.

Two-Wire Macroshock Situations

Two-wire, power-cord-energized equipment that is not double-insulated, and on which the plug is reversible in its receptacle, is extremely hazardous. Unfortunately, much commercial equipment falls into this category. The macroshock situations that can develop with this equipment are illustrated in Figure 2.2.

In part (a) of the figure, a conductive fault has developed between the H lead and the P lead connected to the patient. When the patient completes the circuit by touching the chassis, which is connected to the N lead, the patient receives a hair-raising macroshock. The same thing happens in part (b), except this time the patient completes the circuit by touching the radiator. The radiator is grounded because it is metal and filled with water. The N wire is also attached to ground at the power line service box; this completes the circuit and gives the patient a macroshock. In part (c), the patient is shocked because the plug happens to be reversed in its socket and the H lead gets connected to the chassis that the patient is touching while holding the radiator at the same time, which completes the circuit to ground. In part (d), the patient is in the same position and gets shocked because the H wire has a conductive fault to the chassis. The fuse did not blow out in this case because the N wire is not connected to the chassis, completing the fault circuit to the fuse. In part (e), the patient gets shocked because, with the same kind of conductive fault, the patient completes the circuit between the N wire and the chassis. In part (f), the patient gets shocked because the patient gets across the H wire and the chassis, which is connected to the N wire, completing the circuit through the patient. In part (g), the macroshock is delivered as the patient touches the H wire and ground through the radiator.

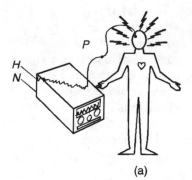

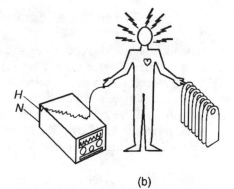

(a)

(b)

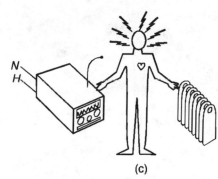

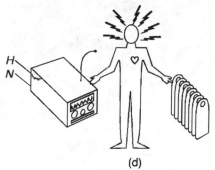

(c)

(d)

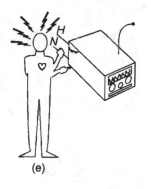

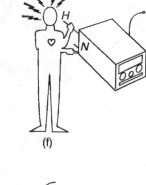

(e)

(f)

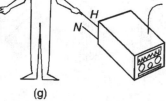

(g)

FIGURE 2.2 Two-wire macroshock situations

Three-Wire Macroshock Situations

Macroshock situations are fewer and more improbable when the equipment has a three-wire plug. Part (a) of Figure 2.3 illustrates a shock being delivered when the H wire and the N wire are touched simutaneously. Likewise, in part (b), the person receiving a macroshock is on the H wire and the grounded chassis. Such situations could result from a frayed power cord. Part (c) illustrates an H wire conductive fault to the chassis that does *not* cause a macroshock because both the chassis

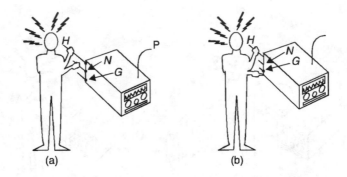

(a)   (b)

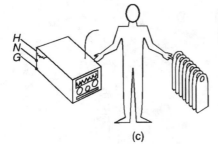
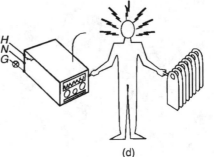

(c)   (d)

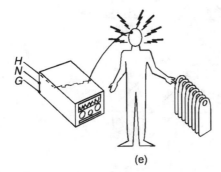
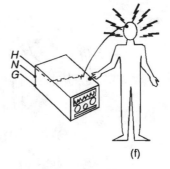

(e)   (f)

FIGURE 2.3   Three-wire macroshock situations

and the radiator are grounded and no potential appears across the person. If such a fault were a short circuit, a circuit breaker would trip, or a fuse would blow out, removing the high voltage from the chassis. In part (d), the same situation as in part (c) only with the G wire also open in a fault results in a macroshock. Notice that two failures had to occur to induce a macroshock in this case, lowering the probability of this happening. In part (e), a conductive fault to a patient lead connected to a patient introduces a macroshock, when the patient touches ground in the radiator. In part (f), the macroshock comes when the patient touches the chassis, which is grounded.

Notice how the three-wire power cord gives more protection against macroshock than the two-wire cord. It protects against conductive faults to the chassis. It also prevents faults due to reversing the plug in the receptacle, because it can be inserted in only one way.

Three-Wire Microshock Situations

In part (a) of Figure 2.4, a microshock affects the patient when leakage from the H wire gets to the P line, either from a stray capacity, dirt, flu-

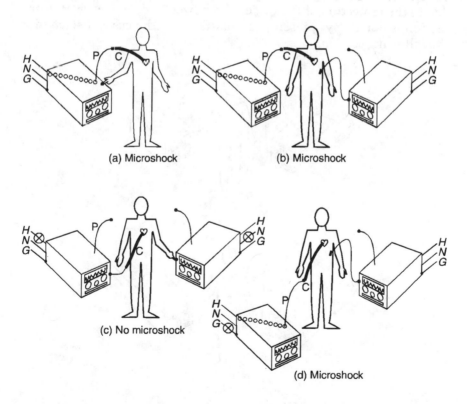

FIGURE 2.4 Three-wire microshock situations

ids, or bad insulation. This leakage current goes directly to the heart through an insulated catheter (C). In this case, the circuit is completed because the patient is contacting the chassis.

In part (b), the leakage current flows through the patient and back to ground through a second instrument. In part (c), the H wire opens on one instrument, and the N wire opens on the other instrument. Microshock does not occur because the power is simply removed by these faults and no excessive leakage current is generated.

In part (d), an open G wire in the instrument on the left causes an increase in P lead leakage and causes a microshock.

The three-wire power cord gives considerable protection against macroshock, but it is not so effective against microshock. One microshock situation that it cures, however, is illustrated in Figure 2.5. In part (a), the patient coming in contact with the two grounded chassis with the two-wire plug receives a microshock because of voltage elevation (as explained in Chapter 1, Example 1.2) due to high current in the N wire. That voltage elevation does not exist in the three-wire case illustrated in part (b) because the G wire does not normally carry a significant current. Thus, the patient does not receive a microshock due to the protection of the three-wire power cord. However, this protection is not always present, as illustrated by the cases discussed in the following section.

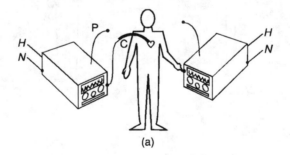

(a)

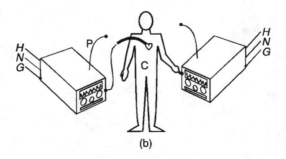

(b)

FIGURE 2.5   How a three-wire plug cures two-wire plug microshock

Attendant-Mediated Microshock

Microshock is insidious because it cannot be felt and leaves no trace in the affected tissue. It is not large enough to stimulate a perceptible number of pain cells to give warning. Therefore, an attendant can pass a microshock to a patient without being aware, except by observing the symptoms of cardiac arrhythmia on the patient.

Any of the microshock situations illustrated in Figure 2.4 could be caused by an attendant who completed the circuit to the source of the shocking current by touching the patient or the patient's catheter. Two such situations are illustrated in Figure 2.6. In part (a), the atten-

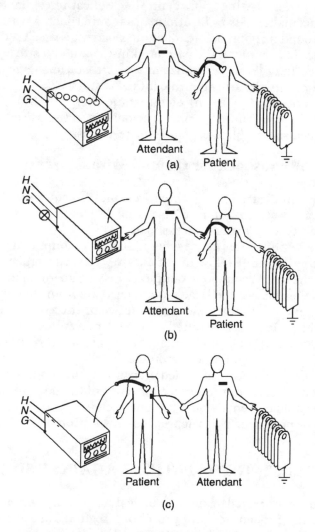

FIGURE 2.6   Attendant-mediated microshock situations

dant completes the circuit to a leaky patient lead by holding it while touching the patient's catheter. In part (b), the attendant completes the circuit by touching a piece of equipment with a voltage elevation due to a faulty power cord. In both cases, the microshock current would pass through the attendant without his or her awareness. Part (c) illustrates the case where the attendant provides the path for the leakage current by touching the patient's body at a place other than the catheter. In this case, the attendant grounds the patient to complete the path for the leakage.

The basic defense of the patient against attendant-mediated microshock is to have the attendant wear insulating gloves whenever touching a patient with a CVC (central vessel catheter), including an external pacemaker. Also, the attendant should touch a water pipe or a known grounding point before touching a patient with a CVC. The attendant should also touch the patient skin-to-skin at a site away from the catheter, in order to neutralize any electrostatic charge on either of them. For example, arm-to-arm contact would work.

This action dissipates any electrostatic charge that may have accumulated. This precaution is made in addition to the use of antistatic garments, bed sheets, blankets, and sterile drapes.

Microshock for Ground Wire Currents

As explained in Figure 2.3, the three-wire plug on equipment protects patients against certain kinds of macroshock. However, it is not as effective in protecting against microshock.

Figure 2.7 illustrates a case where the faulty equipment on the top causes a large current to flow in the G wire. That equipment may not even be in the same room; for example, it may be an air conditioner on the roof. Nevertheless, the large ground currents from that equipment may cause enough voltage elevation between the two devices connected to the patient, as illustrated in part (a), to result in a microshock.

The defense against such microshock is to use a grounding strap between all pieces of equipment grounded to the patient, as illustrated in part (b) of Figure 2.7. As an added precaution, the room may have its own electrical circuit to the service entrance of the power line. In this case, any ground currents would be generated in the room only, where they could be prevented by an appropriate inspection of the equipment.

PROTECTING THE PATIENT AGAINST SHOCK

The patient is protected against electrical hazards by three methods: safe operating procedures and protocols, regular inspection of the equipment, and the use of safety devices. The efficacy of these protec-

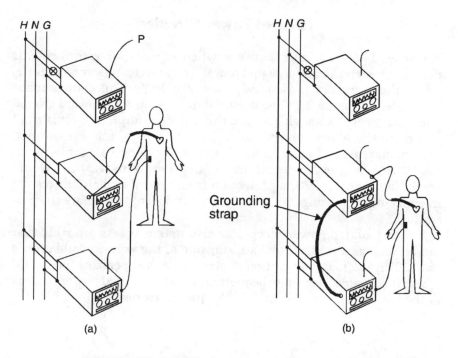

FIGURE 2.7 Grounding strap protection for microshock

tive measures can be illustrated by comparing the safety of commercial airline travel to automobile travel. Although you may feel more vulnerable in an airplane than in an automobile, because an airplane flies in the sky and goes faster, you are safer in an airplane. This is because more rigorous equipment inspections and safety device use are employed on an airplane than in an automobile. Moreover, airplanes are piloted by professionals trained in procedures, whereas automobiles are driven by amateurs who often flaunt the most obvious safety rules. The result is many thousands more fatalities in automobiles per year than in airplanes.

The Three-Prong Plug

The three-prong plug is an effective defense against some macroshock situations. It reduces to low levels voltage elevations between equipment chassis, and it will cause the fuse or circuit breaker to open the circuit in case the H wire shorts to the chassis. Of course, macroshock can still occur in three-wire power cord equipment, as was illustrated in Figure 2.4.

Isolated Power Circuits

An isolated power circuit is created when an isolation transformer is placed between the non-isolated power line and the power receptacle, which thus becomes an *isolated power receptacle*. This connection is illustrated in Figure 2.8. The person touching the *H* wire and ground does not receive a shock because there is no complete circuit from ground to the *N* wire on the isolated (right) side of the transformer. This is macroshock protection. However, if the person got between the *H* wire and the *N* wire on the isolated side, a macroshock would occur. In other words, the protection from an isolated circuit results in a macroshock being less probable, but it doesn't eliminate the possibility.

The isolated power receptacle also makes it less probable that metal, such as a surgical tool striking one of the wires, would draw a spark. This offers fire protection in places like the operating room (OR) where flammable gases may be present. In fact, isolated power circuits in the OR were originally intended for fire protection.

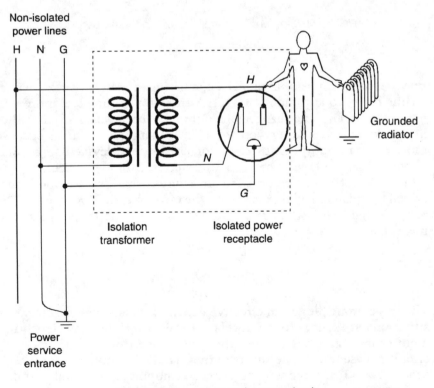

FIGURE 2.8   An isolated power circuit

Line Isolation Monitor

A *line isolation monitor* (LIM) measures how well the H and N leads are isolated from the G wire in an isolated power system. If the isolation deteriorates to the point that a person touching the H wire and ground (as illustrated in Figure 2.8) would draw a dangerous current, an alarm on the LIM would sound. It would sound whether the person was there or not. The alarm does not mean that the dangerous currents are flowing. It merely warns that safety features of the isolation transformer are no longer effective. In a critical situation, such an alarm may often be justifiably ignored.

The alarm on a LIM may be tripped if too many pieces of equipment are attached to the isolated power receptacle. Each added piece of equipment increases the leakage between the N lead and G lead. For example, when enough leakage occurs, a return path from ground to the N lead is established; and the LIM alarm warns of this. In this case, the alarm may be silenced by removing some nonessential equipment.

Ground Fault Interrupter

A *ground fault interrupter* (GFI) protects against macroshock. If more than approximately 3 mA of current flows through a person for more than 200 ms, the GFI will open the circuit and remove the source of macroshock. GFIs are required in wet areas, even in the home in most communities. If, for example, a cord-operated razor fell into the water in the sink, a macroshock would likely result when it is pulled out. The water in the razor would provide a path for the H wire current and shock the person who may be touching the grounded wet sink. However, if a GFI is in place, it would open the circuit and prevent the macroshock.

The GFI circuit in Figure 2.9 consists of the H wire and the N wire being wrapped around a magnetic core. The magnetic field due to the H wire flows opposite to that due to the N wire, and normally these are the same value. This causes the two magnetic fields to cancel each other so that the net magnetic flux is zero. However, if current is flowing to ground in a macroshock situation, such as when the person illustrated in the figure is receiving a macroshock current, the H and N wires will have different current values, and a net magnetic flux will flow in the core and send a signal through the amplifier actuating the relay. This opens the circuit, as illustrated in the figure, and prevents the macroshock from injuring the person.

The GFI looks like an ordinary wall power receptacle, except that it has a reset button. If it is tripped, it should not be reset until a technician has thoroughly checked the circuit for any faults.

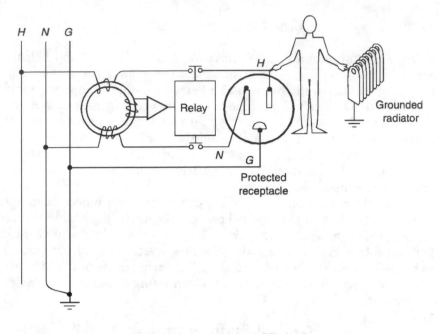

FIGURE 2.9   A tripped GFI circuit

Safety Analyzer

The safety devices discussed thus far help in preventing macroshock, but they are not effective against microshock. The leakage currents are too small to operate protective electronic devices.

When a patient has a central vessel catheter (CVC), one way to protect against microshock is to inspect the equipment used on or near the patient with a safety analyzer. The *safety analyzer* measures the leakage currents from the chassis to ground, from the patient leads to ground, and between patient leads. It measures these currents both when the power cord is normal and when cord faults are simulated.

To measure the leakage currents in a piece of equipment under test (EUT), the power cord of the EUT is plugged into the safety analyzer receptacle, as illustrated in Figure 2.10. The patient leads are connected to the safety analyzer, in accordance with the manufacturer's instructions. The power cord of the safety analyzer is plugged into the wall power receptacle. The leakage currents can then be read on the display. With this safety analyzer, the nurse can plug medical equipment into the analyzer to check for hazardous currents before putting the equipment on a patient. A safety analyzer is illustrated in Figure 2.11.

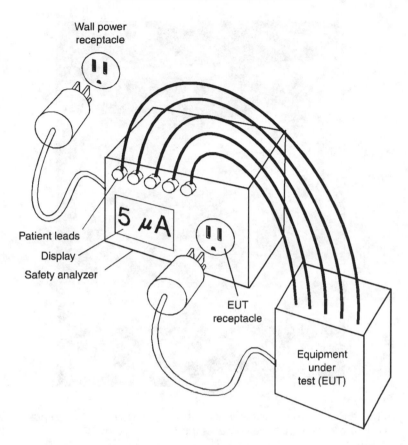

FIGURE 2.10   The safety analyzer

Electrical Safety Inspections

Medical equipment has patient leads that are either *isolated*, measuring many megohms of resistance to the grounded chassis, or *nonisolated*, measuring several kilohms to the chassis. Equipment used when microshock may be a hazard must be isolated. According to the National Fire Protection Association (NFPA, see Klein) the patient leakage currents allowed in isolated equipment are as follows:

Leakage to ground   less than 10 μA
Between leads   less than 10 μA

These limits are required both when the G wire is intact or when it is broken, as simulated by the safety analyzer. The equipment must pass this test both when the power switch is on or when it is off. The chas-

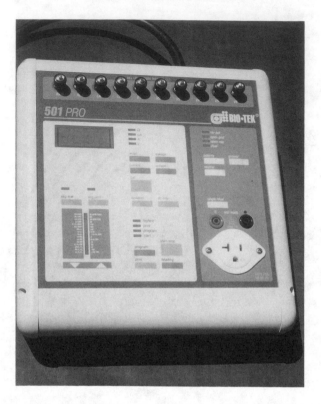

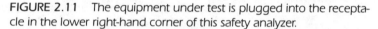

FIGURE 2.11   *The equipment under test is plugged into the receptacle in the lower right-hand corner of this safety analyzer.*

sis leakage to ground when the *G* wire is open must be less than 100 μA in equipment using a power cord.

If the patient leads are non-isolated, the patient lead leakage may be as high as 50 μA. However, this type of equipment may not be used on a patient vulnerable to microshock because of catheters in or near the heart. To minimize voltage elevations on equipment, the resistance between any two exposed metal surfaces may not exceed 0.15 ohms.

The Need for Uninterrupted Power

Many medical instruments, such as ventilators, heart–lung machines, and artificial hearts, serve a continuous life-support function. Power outages, such as those experienced during a thunderstorm, are intolerable in these cases. Just a brief interruption could cause injury or distress to the patient. Most hospitals have an emergency power system, so that power can be restored within ten seconds of a failure of the power mains.

The emergency AC power generator is driven by a gasoline engine. Smaller units may be equipped with batteries that can fill in during these emergencies. Battery operated equipment is more independent of the environment. It can also be safer because the DC current does not cause capacitive and inductive leakage currents. It operates at lower voltages and is isolated from ground, again reducing leakage.

THE OR

The purpose of the operating room (OR) is to provide a theater for the surgeon to give surgical treatments. Every feature should be designed to optimize the procedures while protecting the patient and staff from the environmental hazards. These hazards include infection, electrical shock, toxic materials and gases, ionizing radiation, physical trauma, and fire.

Sterilization

Historically, prevention of infection was the first to receive systematic attention. The OR has a *sterile region*, where the patient, sterile instruments, and surgical staff are located. Aseptic technique requires the surgeons and their staff to scrub their hands and arms. They wear sterile clothing, gloves, gowns, caps, a mask, and shoe covers. The region outside this area is designated as the *unsterile region*, where support personnel and equipment that do not contact the patient are located. Here, personnel dress the same as those in the sterile region, but they do not need to scrub.

The spread of infectious bacteria and viruses is minimized by frequent floor scrubbing and wiping of the walls and equipment. The room is designed to eliminate the spread of microorganisms. Rails for rolling heavy equipment across the ceiling are not recommended. Sliding doors are often used instead of swinging doors, to reduce particulate matter in the air.

Ventilation provides a major defense against the spread of airborne bacteria and toxic gasses. For new construction, 25 changes of air is recommended. This air must come from the outside and be heated. To conserve energy, up to 80 percent of the air is recycled through 0.3 μm filters, which are small enough to eliminate viruses. To prevent the entry of microorganisms from outside the OR, the ventilation fan keeps a positive pressure in the OR; thus the air is always flowing out between the cracks, carrying the microorganisms with it.

Instrument sterilization is done either with steam in an autoclave at high temperature, in ethylene oxide (ETO) at a lower temperature, or with a liquid, such as formaldehyde.

Instruments may be exposed to dry heat at 165° to 170° C for two to three hours. When free-flowing steam is used in an autoclave, a temperature of 144° C for 15 minutes destroys the microorganisms. The instruments are then dried in heated air.

Many instruments, such as plastic implements, electronic pacemakers, and corrosive equipment, cannot withstand the temperature stress of these techniques. Another technique is ETO sterilization, which takes several hours of exposure to the gas at only 60° C. The gas must then be aerated. Since ETO is highly toxic, ventilation is required to ensure the OR does not have more than two parts per million (ppm) present.

Anesthesia

Prior to the 1950s, flammable anesthetics, such as cyclopropane, ethyl ether, ethyl chloride, and ethylene, were commonly used. The flammability of anesthetics is reduced by their combination with a halogen (fluorine, chlorine, or bromine). Thus, the explosive anesthetics have been largely replaced by nonflammables, such as nitrous oxide (N_2O) used in combination with fluorocarbons like methoxyflurane, enflurane, or halothane. Although large concentrations of N_2O can increase the fire hazard, it is a great improvement over the explosive anesthetics; also, endotracheal tubes carrying nonexplosive anesthetic gasses have been ignited by surgical lasers.

An anesthesia machine, as illustrated in Figure 2.12, mixes the anesthetic with O_2 in the proper proportion and delivers it to the patient on a ventilated inspiration cycle. The exhaled gas is cleaned of CO_2 with a soda lime absorber. The gas is vented outside the OR to a suitable collector. In OR ventilation systems that do not recycle and sweep the air out of the exhaust, the anesthetic may be vented into the room. However, these systems waste energy because they have to heat, or cool, much more incoming air than those systems that recycle.

In addition to the ventilation just described, toxic gas safety from the anesthesia machine is ensured by a daily inspection of the machine for low pressure leaks. This is important to eliminate the adverse effects of anesthetics to OR personnel. These include miscarriages, effects on the liver, kidney, and central nervous system, and the increased risk of cancer. The Occupational Safety and Health Administration (OSHA) requires that halogenated anesthetic agents be 2 ppm or less and that N_2O be 25 ppm or less.

Fire Safety

The fire hazard in the OR has been reduced since the 1950s when nonflammable anesthetics were introduced. However, in an enriched oxygen environment, the fire hazard is still appreciable. For example, a fire

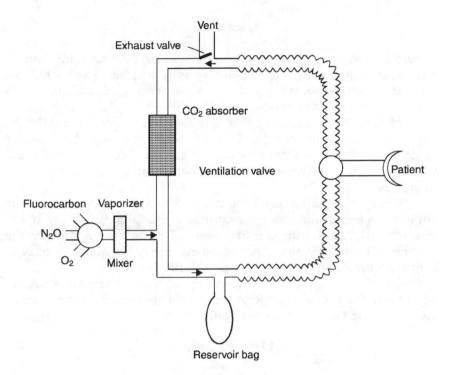

FIGURE 2.12   An anesthesia machine

caused from an electrosurgical scalpel in the vicinity of a leaking oxy-gen tube could occur. Flammable substances found in hospitals include aldehydes, ketones, esters, benzene, toluene, and oils.

One design goal for ORs is to eliminate the sources of sparks and other igniters of fire. Because the flammable gasses and O_2 are heaver than air, and because the ventilator fan pushes air from the ceiling down, the fire hazard is greatest near the floor. To avoid sparks when the plugs are removed, the electrical power receptacles are placed higher than 5 feet above the floor. All hot spots, such as lighting and electronics equipment, should be kept above that level. Fixed lighting is placed 8 feet above the floor.

The isolated electrical system described here is designed to re-duce the probability of sparks. Moreover, the OR floor is electrically conductive, as are the shoes of the personnel. This bleeds off any sta-tic charge buildup that could draw a spark. The resistance of the floor should be less than 5 megohms when measured with an elec-trode 2.5 inches in diameter. To protect the personnel from macroshock, that value should not be less than 10 kohm at any point on the floor. To further prevent sparks, garments and devices should be antistatic.

Gas Safety

Medical gasses, such as oxygen, compressed air, nitrous oxide, and nitrogen, are supplied through pipelines in the hospital. The hazards associated with these are leaks, cross-connecting, unsuspected gas depletion, and contamination.

Misconnections to the gas supply may be avoided by making the pipe size different for each gas. That way the wrong connectors simply will not fit. The consequences of crossed gas lines are serious and could cause anoxia or toxic gas poisoning of a patient on a ventilator or under anesthesia.

Gas contamination can occur when a compressor is used and the input air is contaminated. For example, if the inlet air is near an engine exhaust, bad air can get into the lines. Oil contamination from the compressor motor in the compressed air line could make O_2 or N_2O more flammable when the oil is mixed with them.

Gas leaks of O_2 and N_2O are a fire hazard since they are fire accelerators. They are also toxic in certain concentrations. Large quantities of leaking N_2 can even cause suffocation.

Oxygen Safety

Oxygen is more widely used in the hospital than anesthetics, and may be used in the presence of lesser trained personnel. It presents hazards of fire, pressure trauma, and toxic poisoning.

To prevent the explosion of O_2 containers under as much as 2,100 psig pressure, they should be stored at less than 130° F. That is about the highest temperature at which a person is able to hold onto an oxygen tube without experiencing too much pain. So, as a rule of thumb, if you cannot hold onto an oxygen tube, it is probably too hot.

The O_2 bottles need to be handled carefully so that they are not dropped. If the valves break loose, the jet stream of gas can propel them into objects and personnel, causing physical damage.

Oil and organic gels that may be on a health-care professional's hands must be kept off the oxygen supply valves. These substances and many others, such as human tissue, body oils, silicon rubber, oil-based cosmetics, alcohols, acetone, and epoxy compounds, have increased flammability in an oxygen-rich environment. Personnel and patients around oxygen should remove cosmetics as a precaution. Patient tubing may also be flammable in this environment.

If the valves on the O_2 supply become frozen from low temperature, they should be thawed out and freed with hot, wet rags, rather than with a flame torch. Other sources of ignition, such as matches, burning tobacco, and sparking equipment like portable drills, should be kept away from oxygen.

Hyperbaric Pressure Chambers

In certain surgical procedures, the patient is placed in a high-pressure environment to improve the oxygen transfer properties of the blood. The pressure inside the hyperbaric chamber may be raised to as much as three atmospheres at an oxygen concentration of 100 percent. This allows the use of blood with fewer red blood cells during the operation.

Under these conditions, the danger of a rapidly spreading fire becomes acute. All of the OR precautions designed to prevent fire in the presence of flammable anesthetics must be used. Sources of ignition—electrostatic sparks, sparks from pulling plugs from wall receptacles, nonexplosion-proof foot switches, electronic equipment, portable X rays, cigarette lighters, and the like—must be either eliminated or approved by biomedical engineering. Personnel in this environment should wear fire resistant, antistatic clothing and avoid cotton, wool, synthetic fabrics, and organic cosmetics.

REFERENCES

Aston, R. *Principles of Biomedical Instrumentation and Measurement.* Riverside, N.J.: Macmillan Publishing Company, 1990: Chapter 3.

Carim, H. M. "Bioelectrodes," in *Encyclopedia of Medical Devices and Instrumentation.* Edited by J. G. Webster, New York: John Wiley, 1988, p. 201.

Klein, B. R., ed. *Health Care Facilities Handbook.* 2nd ed. Quincy, Mass.: National Fire Protection Association, 1987.

Laufman, H. *Hospital Special-Care Facilities.* New York: Academic Press, 1981.

Spooner, R. B. *Electrical Safety Simplified.* Englewood Cliffs, N.J.: Prentice-Hall, Inc., 1983.

EXERCISES

1. Prior to what health-care procedure was microshock unknown and not a problem?
2. What is the source of the most recently introduced medical equipment hazard?
3. Above what level of current does microshock occur?
4. Above what level of current does macroshock occur?
5. Why is there no number answer to the question: At what level of voltage does microshock occur?
6. What condition is necessary for microshock to occur, besides a voltage and current being present?

7. Two 1-square-centimeter electrodes are attached to the surface of the body, as illustrated in Figure 2.1. The viscera resistance under the skin is 200 ohms. What will be the total resistance measured between the two electrodes if a conductive gel is used? (The skin-electrode resistance is 10 kΩ.)

8. In exercise 7, what will be the resistance measured between the two electrodes if the area of the electrodes is 10 cm^2 and if a conductive gel is used?

9. In exercise 7, what will be the resistance measured between the two electrodes if the area of the electrodes is 10 cm^2 and if dry electrodes having 100 kΩ/cm^2 resistance are used?

10. Two 15-cm^2 electrodes with a conductive gel are attached to the skin. The viscera resistance is taken as 200 ohms. What is the lowest voltage at which a macroshock will occur in this case?

11. Two 1-square-centimeter dry electrodes are attached to the surface of the skin. The viscera resistance is 200 ohms. If the skin resistance is 100 kΩ, calculate the lowest voltage that could cause a macroshock.

12. In Figure 2.4(a), the resistance between the H lead and the patient lead is 500 kΩ. The catheter, being filled with saline, has a resistance of 50 kΩ. The contact resistance of the patient holding the chassis is 60 kΩ. How much leakage current flows? Does this cause a microshock?

13. In Figure 2.6(a), the resistance due to debris between the H wire and the P lead is 1 megohm. The contact resistance of the hand of the attendant with the P lead is 100 kΩ. The contact of the attendant with the catheter is also 100 kΩ. The patient contact with ground is 50 kΩ. The resistance of the catheter against the heart is 300 ohms. What is the value of leakage current from the 110-volt power line flowing though the patient's heart? Could this cause a microshock?

14. In Figure 2.7(a), the equipment on top has an open N wire. This causes an abnormally high current of 15 A to flow in the G wire. The resistance of the ground wire between the lower two pieces of equipment is 0.15 ohms. What is the value of the voltage elevation between the two chassis?

15. In Figure 2.7(a), the voltage elevation calculated in exercise 14 is applied to the catheter. The significant resistances are a catheter electrode resistance of 200 ohms and a surface contact resistance of 5 kΩ. How much leakage current flows through the patient's heart? Can this current cause a heart ventricular fibrillation (VF)?

16. Describe how the patient connected to the equipment as described in exercise 15 can be protected from a microshock.

17. Why can an attendant cause a microshock in a patient without being aware of it?

18. Why is it difficult to prove that a microshock is the cause of an arrhythmia in a given case?

19. What are the symptoms that a microshock has caused a VF in a patient?

20. What is the defensive action that a nurse should take to protect the CVC patient against microshock when being touched?

21. Describe two ways microshock can be delivered to a patient with a CVC attached to equipment that has an intact G wire.

22. What does the external grounding strap connected between the chassis of two pieces of equipment do to any voltage elevation between them?

23. What is the function of the G wire on the three-prong plug?

24. Why doesn't an isolation transformer eliminate the possibility of receiving a macroshock from an isolated power circuit?

25. What is the function of an LIM?

26. What does the alarm on an LIM warn of?

27. How much current must flow through a GFI in order to cause it to turn the power off?

28. Would a GFI protect a person who touched the N wire with one hand and the H wire with the other hand?

29. If a radio falls into a therapeutic bath and does not touch the patient, would the patient be apt to receive a macroshock?

30. If the patient picks the radio up out of the water, would he or she be apt to get a macroshock?

31. Would a GFI protect the patient in both of these cases, even if the radio did not have a three-prong plug?

32. What is the function of a safety analyzer?

33. Name three paths for leakage that the safety analyzer measures.

34. Which of the following devices is of no help in protecting the patient against microshock?

    (a) three-prong plug   (b) safety analyzer
    (c) GFI   (d) rubber gloves

35. Which of the following is of the most help in protecting the patient against microshock?

    (a) three-prong plug   (b) safety analyzer
    (c) LIM   (d) GFI

36. Name the three most effective means of protecting the CVC patient from microshock.

37. What is the maximum leakage current allowed in normal equipment that has a three-wire power cord and isolated patient leads?

    (a) to ground
    (b) between leads

38. Define patient leads that are

    (a) isolated
    (b) non-isolated

39. Which has fewer paths for leakage current, battery operated equipment or AC powered equipment?

40. How long after the power mains have been interrupted by a power failure must the emergency power system come on line?

41. List four types of hazards in the OR.

42. What technique is required of personnel in the sterile region of the OR, but is not required of personnel in the unsterile region of the OR?

43. What are the two most serious hazards controlled by forced ventilation of the OR?

44. How many changes of air are recommended for newly constructed ORs?

45. What percentage of this air may be recycled?

46. Why does recycling the air save money?

47. Devices to be sterilized in a steam autoclave are raised to what temperature?

48. What is the advantage of ETO sterilization over the autoclave?

49. What is the maximum concentration of ETO allowed in the working environment?

50. Name three major hazards to OR personnel of anesthetic gas leakage.

51. What is the maximum concentration of N_2O allowed in the OR working environment by OSHA?

52. Which of the following protective devices helps the most in eliminating fire-producing sparks from a flammable environment?

    (a) GFI   (b) LIM
    (c) three-prong plug   (d) isolation transformer

53. What feature in the OR helps the most in eliminating electrostatic sparks?

    (a) three-prong plug   (b) conductive floor
    (c) sterile wool drapes   (d) rubber gloves

54. How high must the power receptacles be in an OR checked out for flammable anesthetics?

55. Why are hot devices kept high in an environment where flammable gasses may be present?

56. How are misconnections to the different types of gas lines in a hospital avoided?

57. Name four gasses normally supplied by wall jacks in an OR.

58. What two gasses normally supplied in the hospital wall jacks would be a fire hazard if leaks occurred?

59. Which gas if it leaked would not cause either a fire or a toxic hazard?

60. What is the source of oil contamination in a gas line?

61. What is the highest temperature at which O_2 bottles may be stored?

62. What is the rule of thumb for determining if an O_2 bottle is too hot?

63. What is the proper procedure for freeing a frozen O_2 bottle valve?

64. Name four common materials that have increased flammability in an O_2 environment.

65. What effect does a hyperbaric chamber with an elevated pressure and O_2 concentration have on the patient's blood?

66. What is the highest pressure and O_2 concentration for which a hyperbaric chamber must be certified as fire-safe?

67. Name four types of personal belongings that should not be taken into a hyperbaric chamber.

CHAPTER 3

Transducers, Amplifiers, and Biopotentials

The understanding of how physiological parameters are converted into machine parameters that can be processed into either diagnostic data or therapeutic substances requires that one study the hardware that does this task. Therefore, this chapter begins with a presentation of transducers and amplifiers.

MEDICAL INSTRUMENTATION TRANSDUCERS AND AMPLIFIERS

Transducers in medical instrumentation are crucially important because they come in direct contact with the patient. For this reason, the health-care provider often has primary responsibility for the transducers, the electrodes, and the associated patient leads, cables, tubing, and catheters. Just as it is important that health-care providers understand the psychology and physiology of the patient, it is also important that they understand the physical principles of the transducers and amplifiers that bring diagnostic data from the patient's physiological parameters or that deliver therapeutic substances.

In most cases, the function of the transducer is to convert a physiological parameter—an extremely weak voltage, a pressure, a fluid flow rate, a temperature, a chemical concentration, an electrolyte level—into a voltage that is large enough to be processed accurately by the electronic equipment.

To perform this task, the transducer must be properly placed on the patient, as well as strategically placed into an electronic circuit, such as a Wheatstone bridge (described later in this chapter). Transducer principles are illuminated by the simple and direct analysis of these circuits. This analysis leads to an understanding of transducers and associated equipment interface so that the health-care professional can maximize the accuracy of the data and the safety and comfort of the patient.

A transducer of medical equipment often poses problems for users and maintenance personnel. Because it comes in contact with the patient, safety issues are raised. It is often subject to physical wear and abuse because it is often attached to movable and vulnerable cables. Its performance is often affected by patient motion and tension. Noise and interference factors arise, because the physiological parameters being measured are often very small. Accuracy and calibration become critical, because the data being measured may be used to diagnose disease, prescribe treatment, or deliver therapy.

CONVERSION OF PHYSIOLOGICAL PARAMETERS INTO VOLTAGES

Three of the most commonly measured physiological parameters in health care are temperature, blood pressure, and weight. All of these may be measured by means of a balanced structure, such as a scale. Consider how a scale works. Before the patient steps on it, the scale is in balance, and it reads zero. Another way of saying this is that the scale pointer is on a null. The patient on the scale throws it out of balance, causing a displacement of the pointer, which is calibrated in pounds. In this case, the physiological parameter of weight is transformed to a displacement of a pointer. Here, the transducer is the platform the patient stands on, and the structure of the balance is the arrangement of levers and springs in the scale.

Likewise, the physiological parameters of temperature and pressure are converted to a machine-measurable parameter—voltage—by a balanced structure. In this case, it is a balanced circuit called a Wheatstone bridge.

Wheatstone Bridge

Figure 3.1 illustrates a *Wheatstone bridge,* which consists of four resistors arranged in a diamond shape and labeled R_1, R_2, R_3, and R_X. An excitation voltage, V_E, is applied to two points of the diamond, and an output voltage, V_{OUT}, is measured plus to minus from left to right across the other two points of the diamond. The two resistors on the left, R_X and R_1, form a voltage divider of the V_E excitation. This produces the plus-to-minus voltage drop from node A to

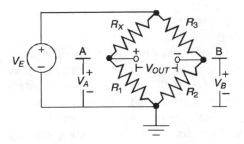

FIGURE 3.1   A Wheatstone bridge

ground, V_A. Likewise, the two resistors on the right, R_2 and R_3, form a voltage divider that creates the voltage drop from node B to ground, V_B.

This circuit can be made balanced, in the simplest case, by making all four resistors the same value. In this case, the voltage divider on the left creates the same voltage as that on the right, because they both have the same excitation voltage and the same resistor values. Thus, V_A equals V_B. The voltage difference between the two nodes is defined as the output voltage, V_{OUT}, so

$$V_{OUT} = V_A - V_B \tag{3.1}$$

In this case, V_{OUT} is zero, and the bridge is said to be at a null point in terms of its resistance values. That is, the bridge is balanced.

This bridge can be made unbalanced by changing the value of R_X. Referring to Figure 3.1, if R_X is caused to increase, the voltage divider on the left will cause V_A to decrease in value. Because the divider on the right is undisturbed, V_B will remain the same. Thus, V_A becomes less than V_B, and V_{OUT}, according to Equation (3.1), becomes a negative voltage. On the other hand, if R_X is caused to decrease from its null value, V_{OUT} will become a positive voltage drop from node A to node B. As an exercise, prove that to yourself by studying the figure.

You have learned the case where the bridge is balanced because all resistors have the same value. In fact, the bridge can be balanced for any number of resistor value combinations given by the formula

$$R_X = R_1 \frac{R_3}{R_2} \tag{3.2}$$

This equation is called the *null condition* for the bridge. For the bridge configuration shown in Figure 3.1, if R_X is increased above the value given by this equation, V_{OUT} will leave zero and be a negative voltage. And if R_X is decreased from its null value, V_{OUT} will become positive. A derivation for Equation (3.2) is given in the Appendix, Section A.2.

Thermistor

A *thermistor* is a transducer that makes it possible to convert the physiological parameter of temperature into a voltage. A thermistor may be constructed of a cube of material, about 0.1 inch on a side, embedded in glass whose electrical resistance varies with its temperature. Almost all electrical conductors exhibit this property to some degree. For example, if copper is heated, the atoms will vibrate harder, making it more difficult for free electrons to get past without a collision. This increases its resistance. Thus, copper has a *positive temperature coefficient*, because an increase in temperature causes an increase in resistance. Some metals act similarly, but in the opposite direction. For example, an increase in temperature in a semiconducting metal like silicon will break more electrons free from their crystal bonds and increase the number of free electrons, so that an increase in temperature will decrease the resistance. Because of this, silicon is said to have a *negative temperature coefficient*. Commonly used thermistor elements are made from oxides of nickel, copper, or aluminum. This gives the thermistor elements a relatively high temperature coefficient.

Temperature Transducer

A thermistor mounted in a Wheatstone bridge can function as the transducer that converts body temperature to a voltage. This may be used as the transducer for an electronic thermometer. Its advantage over the traditional mercury thermometer is its fast response time and ease of reading, not to mention the fact that mercury from a broken thermometer is a hazardous material. In a blood donor screening, for example, reducing the three minutes it takes to do a temperature with a mercury thermometer becomes important. On the other hand, the electronic thermometer is more complicated, bulkier, and may not last as long as the mercury thermometer.

Pressure Transducer

Blood pressure is most commonly measured with an air cuff and stethoscope using a device called a *sphygmomanometer*. This is the noninvasive test given in a blood donor screening. For intensive care situations, however, it may be necessary to use an invasive procedure. The details of these procedures are explained in Chapter 9. Here, the focus is on how the physiological parameter of pressure is transformed into a voltage.

A commonly used pressure transducer is shown in Figure 3.2. The dome on the top may be filled with a saline solution that articulates to a catheter, as in the heart to measure the blood pressure in a ventricle. The other fluid coupling connection is blocked off. Changes in

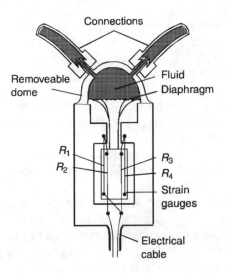

FIGURE 3.2   A pressure transducer

blood pressure propagate through the catheter and cause small displacements in the diaphragm. These displacements move a plunger to which are connected four wires, called *strain gauges*. With each displacement, two of these wires lengthen and the other two get shorter. Lengthening the wire increases its resistance, while shortening the wire decreases its resistance by the same amount. [The formula for resistance in Equation (1.1) shows that lengthening a wire causes it to increase in resistance both because it gets longer and because its cross-sectional area reduces.] These high resistance wires are arranged in the form of a Wheatstone bridge, as shown in Figure 3.3.

   In the figure, each of the strain gauge wires is represented by a resistor, R, plus a change in resistance, ΔR, imposed by changes in pressure on the diaphragm. Notice on the left branch of the bridge that a positive ΔR increases the upper resistance and decreases the lower resistance. Thus, V_A would decrease. Because of the change in sign of the ΔRs on the right branch, V_B would go in the opposite direction and increase. The net result is that V_{OUT}, defined as plus to minus from node A to node B, would be a negative voltage. If the pressure on the diaphragm changes to the opposite direction, V_{OUT} would become a positive voltage. Thus, you have a mechanism that converts the pressure

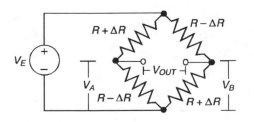

FIGURE 3.3   A pressure transducer circuit

changes into voltage changes. This voltage could be used to drive electrical meters and monitoring equipment.

Pressure Transducer Sensitivity

In general, the *sensitivity* of a pressure transducer, S_V, is defined as the change in output voltage per volt of excitation per millimeter of mercury of applied pressure (V/V/mmHg).

A typical commercially available pressure transducer has a sensitivity ranging from 5 μV/V/mmHg to 40 μV/V/mmHg, depending upon the manufacturer and model.

Some *disposable pressure transducers* work on the same electrical principle just described. The manufacturing process for these transducers is inexpensive enough that the unit can be disposed of rather than put through an expensive sterilization process. In fact, in some cases, trying to sterilize a disposable unit can damage it and make it inaccurate.

VOLTAGE AMPLIFIERS

Amplifiers are older than history. A lever with a fulcrum for prying up stone is a force amplifier. A force down on one side of the lever will cause a larger force going in the opposite direction to be exerted on the other side of the lever. The closer the fulcrum is to what is being pried up, the larger that force will be. Notice that the output force is in the opposite direction from the input force. This is an example of an *inverting amplifier.*

A pressure amplifier is illustrated in Figure 3.4. It consists of two disks attached to either end of a rod. If a pressure is exerted on the

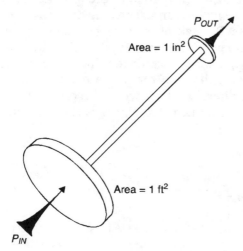

P_{OUT}

Area = 1 in²

Area = 1 ft²

P_{IN}

FIGURE 3.4   A pressure amplifier

larger disk in the direction shown in the figure, the smaller disk will exert a larger pressure in the same direction. For example, if P_{IN} on the disk on the left is 1 pound per square foot on a 1-square-foot area, the rod will transmit that 1 pound to the smaller disk at a pressure of 1 pound per square inch. This converts to a pressure of 144 pounds per square foot. This, therefore, is an example of a pressure amplifier with a gain of 144. In this case, the output pressure, P_{OUT}, is in the same direction as P_{IN}. This is an example of a *noninverting amplifier.*

The tympanic membrane and the oval window of the inner ear form a pressure amplifier of this type.

Differential Amplifier

The surface potentials that are measured on the body for medical diagnosis, such as the electrocardiogram (ECG), the electroencephalogram (EEG), and the electromyogram (EMG), are all difference potentials. A *difference potential* is that voltage measured between two sites on the body. For example, the ECG measured between two wrists is a difference potential. The amplifier for measuring difference potentials is called a *differential amplifier.* To make a differential amplifier, electronic transistors are arranged in the form of a Wheatstone bridge.

A differential amplifier, often abbreviated as *diff amp*, is an electronic amplifier in which the output voltage is proportional to the difference between two input voltages. Diff amps are particularly useful for measuring biopotentials, because many biopotentials of clinical and medical diagnostic significance consist of the difference in voltage on two body sites. The EEG is the difference in surface potential between two skull sites. Likewise, the EMG records the difference between two potentials measured on a muscle. The diff amp is ideal for measuring these difference potentials and is often used in medical instrumentation.

The Ideal Diff Amp Concept

The ideal diff amp is an elegant and powerful concept. It helps explain a large number of medical instrumentation principles and is used often in the remainder of this text.

A diff amp is defined as an electronic amplifier in which the output voltage, V_{OUT}, is proportional to the difference between the two input voltages, V_1 and V_2. This definition can be written mathematically as

$$V_{OUT} = A_D (V_2 - V_1) \qquad (3.3)$$

where A_D is the gain of the amplifier. The schematic symbol for the diff amp, given in Figure 3.5, shows the orientation of the parameters of

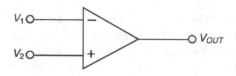

FIGURE 3.5   Diff amp schematic symbol

this equation. V_1, measured from plus to minus to ground from the upper input node, is the inverting input voltage. V_2, measured to ground from the lower input node, is the noninverting input voltage. The gain, A_D, is the ratio of the output voltage to the difference between the two input voltages. It is a dimensionless number.

This will be considered an ideal diff amp when the resistance at each input node is very large (more than 40 megohms). This means that essentially zero current will flow into either of the input nodes. Another implication is that attaching the input leads of the diff amp to another circuit will not disturb that circuit in any way. In measuring body surface potentials, for example, this would imply that attaching the amplifier to the sites measured would not distort those voltages, introduce artifacts, or attenuate them. In other words, the ideal diff amp is "invisible" to the parameter it measures. In the ideal diff amp, the V_{OUT} measured to ground is given by Equation (3.3), and the output resistance approaches zero. This means that the load placed on the output of the amplifier will not change the value of the output, V_{OUT}.

In Equation (3.3), notice that when the input voltages, V_1 and V_2, are the same (or *common-mode*), the output voltage is zero. This is what is meant when a diff amp is said to reject common-mode voltage. In other words, the output due to a common-mode voltage at the inputs is zero in an ideal diff amp.

Common-Mode Voltage Interference

The importance of diff amps is heightened by the fact that one of the major tasks in monitoring, diagnosing, and making measurements on medical patients is the measurement of difference potentials that occur in the body; that is, the ECG, EEG, or EMG. They are all measured as differences between sites on the surface of the body. In each case, the instrument for doing this is the diff amp.

The situation in making a difference measurement on the body is shown in Figure 3.6. This illustrates the basic problem of such a measurement in the hospital environment—power line, 60-cycle interference. In such an environment, where thousands of pieces of electrical equipment are in use, the power requirements are high. Inevitably, patients are in close proximity to power buses through stray capacity be-

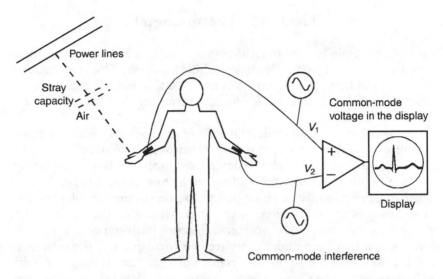

FIGURE 3.6 Power line interference in biopotential measurements

tween them and their bodies, which are essentially conductors. The amount of capacity is in the order of 10 pF (10×10^{-12} farad). This value varies widely with the situation, but it should give you a feeling for how much capacity is involved. This capacity couples a current into the patient and generates a voltage on the input terminals V_1 and V_2 in Figure 3.6.

The value of the voltages is the same on both terminals because the body is all one conductor. Therefore, the voltages are common-mode voltages. A common-mode voltage is one that has the same value over the entire surface of the body. The value of the voltages is about 2 volts at 60 cycles. You can measure these voltages on an oscilloscope by simply holding onto the conducting end of the input lead. They are much larger in size than the body potential voltages of an ECG, which is about 1 mV. Because they are common-mode voltages fed to a diff amp, the diff amp output due to them is ideally zero. However, the output due to the ECG will be whatever its difference value is at the input multiplied by the gain, A_D. That is, the diff amp rejects the common-mode 60-cycle voltage, but it passes the difference potentials under test.

Real world diff amps are not ideal, so they do not perfectly reject common-mode voltage interference. For them, the *common-mode rejection ratio* (CMRR) is defined as the ratio of the V_{OUT} due to a voltage when presented to the amplifier as a common-mode signal to the V_{OUT} due to the same signal presented as a difference voltage. This CMRR is often given in decibels (dB) and would have a value in excess of 100 dB in a useful diff amp.

Electronic Thermometer

A simple example of how the diff amp is used in a medical instrument is as a component of an electronic thermometer. The temperature transducer defined previously can be used along with a diff amp to make such a thermometer. A block diagram of the thermometer is shown in Figure 3.7.

In order to have an understanding of this device, or any medical instrument for that matter, it is important to be able to follow the information variables through the device, beginning with the physiological parameter under test and ending with the output display data. In Figure 3.7, temperature, T, is applied to the thermometer. The temperature changes the resistance in the thermistors in the bridge. This determines the value of the voltage difference between nodes (connections) A and B. These nodes are wired to the diff amp, the output of which is proportional to the difference voltage. That voltage then drives the display on the scale where a number corresponding to the temperature appears.

Pressure Monitor

A pressure monitor uses a diff amp in a similar fashion. In both cases, it responds to the voltage developed across the output of a Wheatstone bridge and drives a display. The elements of a pressure monitor are

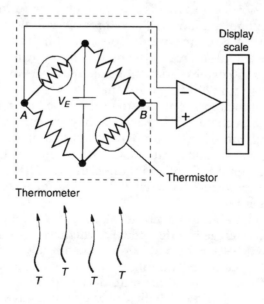

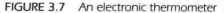

FIGURE 3.7   An electronic thermometer

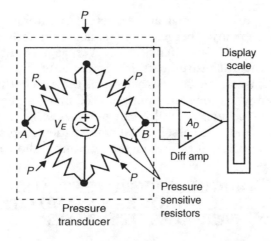

FIGURE 3.8 A blood pressure monitor

shown in Figure 3.8. The path of the information variables of pressure, *P*, and voltage through the instrument is as follows: The pressure from the fluid catheter in the blood vessel is exerted on the pressure-sensitive resistors in the Wheatstone bridge. The difference voltage from nodes *A* to *B* that results is wired to the diff amp, which produces a voltage output proportional to it. The output from the diff amp drives the display unit, which gives a reading of the pressure.

This is essentially the process that occurs both for many reusable and disposable pressure transducer-driven monitors. Figure 3.8 just illus-

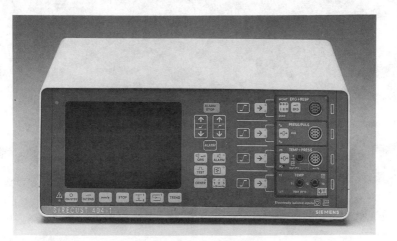

FIGURE 3.9 A monitor for pressure, temperature, and the electrocardiogram (Courtesy of Siemens Medical Systems, Inc.)

trates the conceptual block diagram. An actual monitor in use in the hospital would have many other features to ensure reliability, ease of use, accuracy, safety, and convenience. However, as part of the process of learning about medical instruments, it is important to memorize the conceptual block diagram and be able to describe the path of the information variables. Then when the instrument is used in a complex therapeutic and diagnostic procedure, the health-care provider will manipulate it with more confidence and in the best interest of the patient. A practical unit for monitoring patient ECG pressure and temperature is shown in Figure 3.9.

ORIGIN OF BIOPOTENTIALS, ELECTROCARDIOGRAMS, AND OTHER SURFACE POTENTIALS*

The biopotential was scientifically investigated as early as 1786 by Luigi Galvani, an Italian physicist. His studies led to the invention of the voltaic cell by another Italian physicist, Count Miessandro Volta.

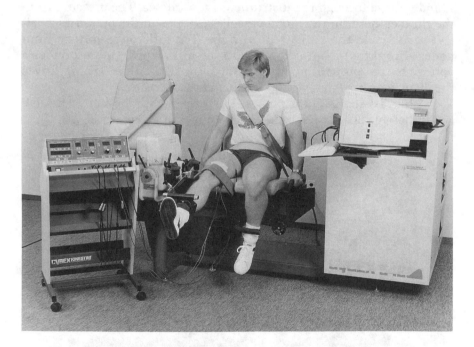

FIGURE 3.10   Monitoring biopotentials. (Courtesy of Cybex Division of Lumex)

*This section is reprinted with permission of Merrill, an imprint of Macmillan Publishing Company, from *Principles of Biomedical Instrumentation and Measurements*, by Richard Aston, copyright 1990 by Macmillan Publishing Company.

The process in the body that produces biopotentials is very similar to the process that produces the voltage in a conventional battery; hence, the following definition: A *biopotential* is an electrical voltage caused by a current flow of ions through biological tissue.

The study of biopotentials is fundamental to the understanding of medical instrumentation. Several of the major types of equipment, including electrocardiographs and electroencephalographs, measure biopotentials from the surface of the body. Physicians use the data obtained from these instruments to assess the health of their patients. A patient having his biopotentials monitored is shown in Figure 3.10.

All people who work with medical instrumentation must understand the safety issues associated with biopotentials. The primary hazard is electrical shock, which was discussed in Chapters 1 and 2.

BIOPOTENTIALS

The single cell is the unit from which living systems are built. Its complexity is illustrated by the fact that within its membrane occur hundreds of chemical reactions, many of which are not understood. You can observe a membrane potential, V_m, in living cells by inserting a microtip-wire or a conductor-filled glass electrode into the cell, as shown in Figure 3.11. The measured value of V_m is usually in the order of –90 mV.

The potential appearing across the cell membrane is the basis for the biopotentials measured on the body, such as the electrocardiogram

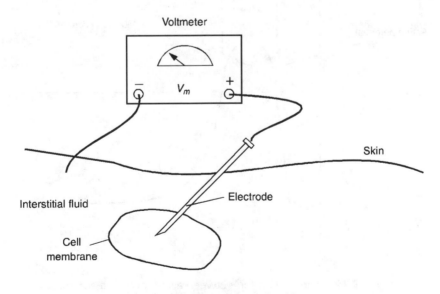

FIGURE 3.11 Measuring V_m

(ECG), electroencephalogram (EEG), electrooculogram, electroretino-gram, or electromyogram (EMG). Notice that the suffix *gram*, as in electrocardiogram, designates the potential itself, whereas the suffix *graph*, as in electrocardiograph, designates the instrument that measures or records the potential (Aston, pp. 37–39).

Action Potential and Muscle Contraction

Living cells are encased with a high-resistance membrane, which, at rest, has a potential caused by the flow of sodium and chlorine ions into the cell and the flow of potassium ions out of it. The resting potential, V_m, typically has values between –50 mV and –100 mV. If the potential is raised across the membrane by about 20 percent, a stimulus threshold is exceeded and the cell membrane resistance changes, causing a change in the membrane potential. This new membrane potential, called *action potential*, is shown in Figure 3.12. While the action potential exists, the cell is said to be *depolarized* (Aston, p. 44). After a period of time (8 ms in Figure 3.12), the membrane resistance will return to its rest value, the membrane will *repolarize*, and the membrane potential will return to its resting potential, V_m, as well. In some tissue, this process may take as long as 300 ms.

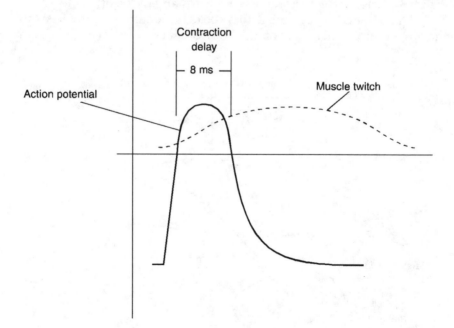

FIGURE 3.12   The relationship between action potential and muscle contraction

In tissue, the depolarization of one cell will stimulate depolarization in an adjacent cell, causing a propagation of the depolarization throughout the tissue, as illustrated in Figure 3.13. In part (a), the tissue is polarized. Then a stimulus, whether it be mechanical, chemical, or electrical, causes one cell to depolarize. This means that the region around the cell is negative, while the rest of the tissue is relatively positive. This causes an ionic current, I, to flow from the positive region to the negative region. That current then stimulates the adjacent cell to depolarize, as illustrated in part (c). That generates more I stimulating other adjacent cells until the entire tissue is depolarized, as illustrated in part (e). At this point, the I goes to zero because there is no potential difference in the interstitial fluid.

By this time, the first cell is ready to repolarize and return to its rest state, as illustrated in part (f). This causes I to flow in the opposite direction. Repolarization then propagates throughout the tissue, as illustrated in parts (g) and (h), until the tissue is fully polarized, as illustrated in part (i). The I again reduces to zero, and the cells in the tissue remain in the rest state.

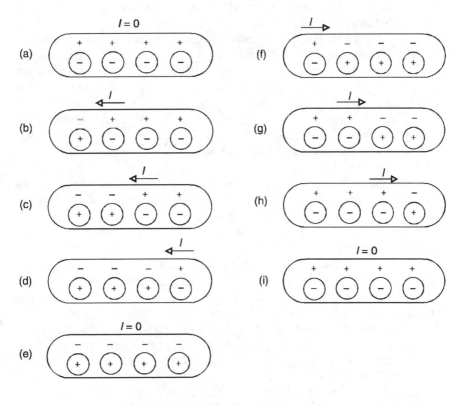

FIGURE 3.13   The depolarization process

In muscle, the cells are situated in an orderly arrangement. Thus, when the depolarized cell creates the positive charge in its vicinity, an attractive force is applied to an adjacent cell, so that the cells move toward each other. This causes the tissue to contract. When this occurs throughout the muscle, it is known as a *muscle contraction*. This contraction process takes some time. For example, a muscle twitch or displacement is observed in Figure 3.12 to occur about 8 ms after the action potential has passed in one of the cells. The observed muscle twitch is the result of many cells acting together.

A stimulus voltage generally does not affect a cell while it is changing its polarization. The *refractory period* is the duration of a cell's nonresponse to further stimuli. During the *relative refractory period*, a higher stimulus is required to reinitiate an action potential and the subsequent contraction of muscle (Aston, p. 45).

Biopotentials in the Heart

The electrical activity of the heart is integral to the operation of several types of medical instruments, including the electrocardiograph, pacemaker, and defibrillator. Very small electrical disturbances can cause this vital organ to cease pumping the blood necessary to sustain life.

The heart consists of two major smooth muscles, the atrium and the ventricle, which form a syncytium, or fusion of cells, that conducts depolarization from one cell to the adjacent one. Because of ionic leakage in the smooth muscle membrane, the tissue of the heart does not require an external stimulus; rather, it depolarizes spontaneously from its resting state and effectively oscillates, or beats. The sinoatrial (SA) node beats from 70 to 80 beats per minute (bpm) at rest; the atrioventricular (AV) node beats at 40 to 50 bpm, and the bundle branches oscillate at 15 to 40 bpm.

The SA node normally determines the heart rate, because it beats at the fastest rate and causes stimulation of the other tissue before it reaches its self-pacing threshold. Thus, the SA node can be considered the heart's pacemaker. The path of the depolarization of cells in a heart is illustrated in Figure 3.14.

The depolarization of the SA node spreads throughout the atrium and reaches the AV node in about 40 ms. Because of the low conduction velocity of the AV node tissue, it requires about 110 ms for the depolarization to reach the bundle branches, called the *purkinje system*. The ventricles then contract. The right ventricle forces blood into the lungs, and the left ventricle pushes blood into the aorta and subsequently through the circulation system. The contraction period of the heart is called *systole*.

The action potentials in the ventricle hold from 200 to 250 ms. This relatively long time allows the ventricular contraction to empty

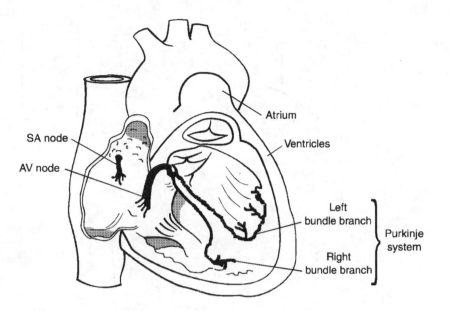

FIGURE 3.14   *The depolarization path through the heart (Reprinted by permission of Macmillan Publishing Company)*

blood into the arteries. The heart then repolarizes during a rest period called *diastole*. Then the cycle repeats.

THE ELECTROCARDIOGRAM

During diastole, all of the cells are polarized so that the potential inside each cell is negative with respect to the outside. Normally, depolarization occurs first at the SA node, making the outside of the tissue negative with respect to the inside of the cells as well as to the tissue not yet depolarized. This imbalance results in an ionic current, I, causing the left arm to measure positive with respect to the right arm, as illustrated in Figure 3.15(a). The resulting voltage is called the *P wave*. After about 90 ms, the atrium is completely depolarized, and the ionic current measured by lead I reduces to zero. The depolarization then passes through the AV node, causing a delay of about 110 ms. The depolarization then passes into the right ventricular muscle, depolarizing it and causing it to be negative relative to the still-polarized left ventricular muscle, as illustrated in Figure 3.15(b). Again, the direction of I causes a plus-to-minus voltage from the left arm to the right arm called the *R wave*. Repolarization of the heart causes the T wave as shown in Figure 3.15(c).

The complete waveform in Figure 3.16 is called an *electrocardiogram* (ECG), with the labels *P, Q, R, S,* and *T* indicating its distinctive

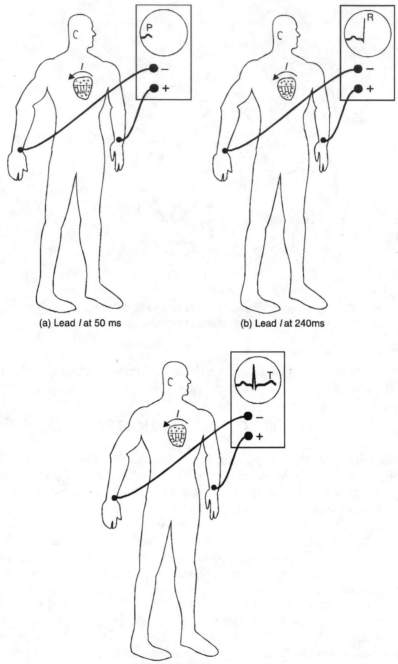

(a) Lead I at 50 ms   (b) Lead I at 240ms

(c) Lead II at 450 ms

FIGURE 3.15   Relating ECG to heart electrical activity. (Reprinted by permission of Macmillan Publishing Company)

features. The *P* wave arises from depolarization of the atrium. The *QRS* complex arises from depolarization of the ventricles. The magnitude of the *R* wave within this complex is approximately 1 mV. The *T* wave arises from repolarization of the ventricle muscle. During the *T* wave, partial repolarization of the cardiac muscle causes an ionic current, and a corresponding ECG potential, as was described for the *R* wave. The *U* wave, which sometimes follows the *T* wave, is a second-order effect of uncertain origin and is of little diagnostic significance. The intervals, segments, and complexes of the ECG are defined in Figure 3.16. Typical durations are as follows:

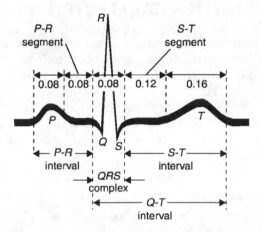

Intervals:

P-R . . . Beginning of *P* wave to beginning of *QRS* complex

S-T . . . End of *S* wave to end of *T* wave

Q-T . . . Beginning of *Q* wave to end of *T* wave

Segments:

P-R . . . End of *P* wave to beginning of *Q* wave

S-T . . . End of *S* wave to beginning of *T* wave

Complex:

QRS . . . Beginning of *Q* wave to end of *S* wave

Durations:

Average durations shown on drawing, in seconds

FIGURE 3.16   An EGC (Courtesy of Hewlett-Packard Company)

FEATURE	DURATION (ms)
QRS complex	60 to 100
R–R interval	600 to 1000
P–R interval	120 to 200

The *QRS* duration, *P–R* interval, and *S–T* interval depend on the depolarization rate of the heart. The ranges shown here reflect the individual differences seen in a normal population (Aston, pp. 45–49).

BIOPOTENTIAL ELECTRODES

An electrode transducer couples the voltage on the surface of the body to an electronic instrument. The surface potentials on the body range from 1 microvolt (μV) on the skull to 1 millivolt (mV) across the arms to a 0.1 V on exposed viscera. The electrodes are either *invasive*, as in the case of a needle electrode that penetrates the skin, or *noninvasive*, as in surface electrodes that do not penetrate the skin. The most frequently encountered type of electrode used in the clinical environment is the surface electrode.

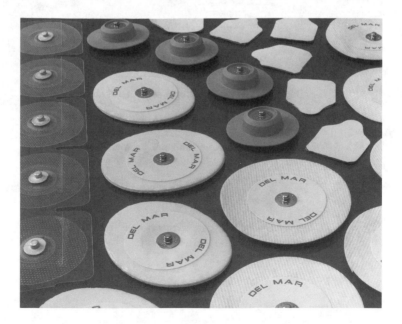

FIGURE 3.17   *These disposable electrodes range from conductive adhesive tabs (1) to pre-gelled adhesive electrodes (2). (Courtesy of Delmar Avionics)*

Surface Electrode

The surface electrode may consist of a metal plate coated with an electrolyte solution. Sometimes, though, it may be formed by a metal plate separated from the surface of the body by an insulator, thereby forming a capacitive coupling (Aston, p. 90). Two types of metal surface electrodes are the suction electrode, which can be readily moved about and is held in place against the skin by suction, and the metal surface electrode, which is attached to a limb using the elastic band. Both of these electrodes require an electrolyte gel interface with the skin.

An assortment of disposable adhesive electrodes is shown in Figure 3.17. A conductive adhesive electrode is labeled (1) in the figure.

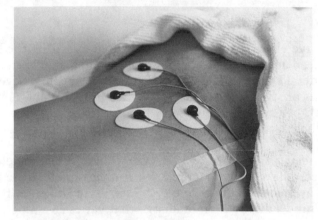

(a)

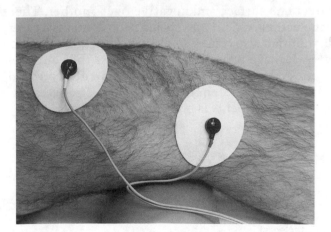

(b)

FIGURE 3.18   (a) Pre-gelled disposable electrodes; (b) a surface electrode (Courtesy of Consolidated Medical Corporation)

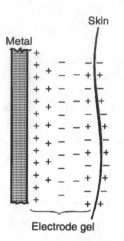

Skin

Metal

Electrode gel

FIGURE 3.19   The charge distribution of a surface electrode

The adhesive electrode labeled (2) is formed by filling the hole in a donut-shaped adhesive tape surrounding a metal snap with electrode gel. The metal snap attaches to an electrode lead cable. Several common means of attaching the electrodes are illustrated in Figure 3.18. In part (a), pre-gelled electrodes for measuring any potential are shown attached to the back. Larger electrodes are attached to the leg in part (b).

To understand the principle of operation of the metal-electrolyte surface electrode, consider Figure 3.19. A metal-to-electrode potential is formed by electrons that leave the electrolyte and enter the metal, leaving behind a distribution of charge that varies as a function of position. This charge distribution is similar to that of a capacitor: it is positive over one surface and negative over another. Therefore, the equivalent electrical circuit for this junction contains a capacitor. This charge distribution also causes an electric potential called the *half-cell potential*. A leakage resistance exists across the equivalent capacitance. A series resistance in the equivalent circuit represents the electrolyte fluid in charge equilibrium. The arrangement of these equivalent circuit elements is given in Figure 3.20.

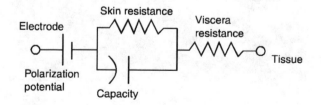

FIGURE 3.20   Equivalent circuit of a surface electrode

REFERENCES

Aston, R. *Principles of Biomedical Instrumentation and Measurement.* Columbus, Ohio: Charles E. Merrill Publishing Company, 1990.

Clark, J. W. "The Origin of Biopotentials." Chapter 4 in *Medical Instrumentation, Applications and Design.* Edited by J. G. Webster. Boston: Houghton Mifflin, 1978.

Floyd, T. L. *Electronic Devices.* Columbus, Ohio: Charles E. Merrill Publishing Company, 1984.

Guyton, A. C. "The Heart." Part III of *Textbook of Medical Physiology.* 3rd ed. Philadelphia: W. B. Saunders, 1966.

EXERCISES

1. Give three reasons why it is important for a nurse to understand medical instrumentation transducers.

2. What is the function of a transducer?

3. Why is an amplifier necessary in equipment that monitors biopotentials?

4. List three factors that commonly cause problems with transducers.

5. List three types of problems that you may encounter in transducers.

6. List three commonly measured physiological parameters that require a transducer to convert them to a voltage.

7. Referring to Figure 3.1, write the condition for balance in the Wheatstone bridge.

8. Referring to Figure 3.1, assume that $R_1 = 5$ kohm, $R_2 = 15$ kohm, and $R_3 = 10$ kohm. What must the value of R_X be in order to make V_{OUT} equal 0 V?

9. Referring to Figure 3.1, assume that $V_E = 10$ V, $R_X = 20$ kohm, and the values of R_1, R_2, and R_3 are the same as in Exercise 8. Calculate the new value of V_{OUT}.

10. Define a negative temperature coefficient.

11. Explain why copper has a positive temperature coefficient.

12. Name two advantages and two disadvantages of an electronic thermometer over a mercury thermometer.

13. Why would two thermistors instead of one be placed in a Wheatstone bridge to make a temperature transducer?

14. Does the resistance of a copper wire increase or decrease when you stretch it? Explain why.

15. Why could you call a lever an inverting amplifier?

16. Suppose that in Figure 3.4, P_{IN} equals 5 psi. What is the output, P_{OUT}?

17. Suppose that in Figure 3.4, P_{IN} equals 10 mmHg. What will be the pressure out, P_{OUT}?

18. State the definition of a diff amp.

19. In a diff amp, suppose that the voltage at the inverting input is 5 V and the voltage at the noninverting input is 3.5 V. If the differential gain is 12, what is the value of V_{OUT}?

20. What is the input resistance of an ideal diff amp?

21. How much current does an ideal amplifier draw from the circuit that delivers an information variable to it.

22. Sketch the block diagram of an electronic thermometer.

23. Describe the path of the information variables through the electronic thermometer in Figure 3.7.

24. Draw a block diagram of an electronic blood pressure monitor.

25. Describe the path of the information variables through the pressure monitor in Figure 3.8.

26. Why is a disposable pressure transducer economically viable?

CHAPTER 4

The Electrocardiograph

Next to the primary-care instruments, such as the scale, thermometer, and sphygmomanometer, the electrocardiograph is the most common. That's because the screening test takes less than ten minutes, has simple, painless limb lead connections, and is done with readily available instrumentation found in most health-care facilities.

The *electrocardiograph* (ECG) is an electronic instrument that measures the surface potentials appearing between two limbs of the body. These potentials, or voltages, arise from the electrical activity of the heart. The initials *ECG* are also used to identify the *electrocardiogram,* which is the graphical record of these potentials as a function of time. The exact meaning of *ECG* is usually clear from the context.

LEAD CONNECTIONS

The measurement technique for ECGs in its simplest form is illustrated in Figure 4.1(a). Here, the physiological information parameter is the biopotential difference between the two arms. The potential on each limb is directly connected through a biopotential electrode to the two inputs of a differential amplifier. This amplifier produces an output voltage amplified in proportion to that biopotential difference. That voltage then drives the display unit, which records the ECG signal as a function of time.

That explains the information path from the heart to the display; but to understand how to get the most diagnostic information out of the heart's electrical activity, many more details need to be considered.

First, the effects of the skin resistance and polarization potential, E_p, of the electrodes should be considered. An equivalent circuit illustration of how these are related to the equipment is shown in part (b) of Figure 4.1. If both electrodes are identical and connected in the same fashion to the skin, the E_p would be identical on both terminals and

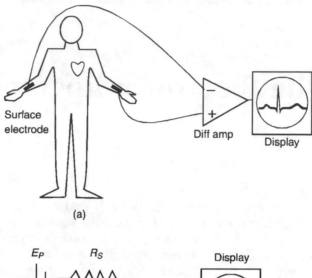

(a)

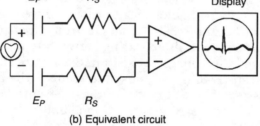

(b) Equivalent circuit

FIGURE 4.1　Information flow in the ECG test

would therefore produce a zero output voltage from the differential amplifier. In that way, the differential amplifier cancels the effect of polarization voltage. Because this potential stays the same, while the ECG from the heart varies as a function of time, one can compensate for it on the display by an offset adjustment in case the electrode connections are not identical.

However, if the patient moves and disturbs the electrode connection, the distribution of ions in the electrolyte would also be changed. The corresponding change in E_p would show up as a slow motion of the ECG signal reference, called a *baseline wander*. This is illustrated in part (a) of Figure 4.10, page 101. When a cold electrode is first applied to the skin, it will tend to warm up to body temperature. This, too, may affect the polarization potential. These problems can be corrected by asking the patient to stop moving or by tightening or changing the electrode connections to the skin, or by waiting for temperature equilibrium.

Another kind of interference occurs in the ECG trace because of the 60-cycle alternating (AC) current in the power lines. Figure 4.2 il-

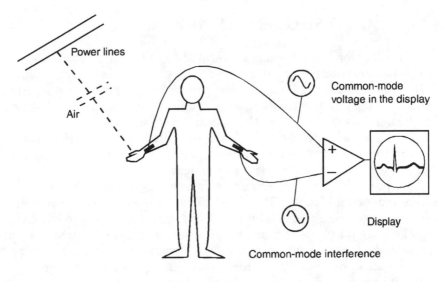

FIGURE 4.2 ECG AC interference

lustrates how the patient receives current from the power lines through capacitive coupling to them. A capacitor is formed whenever two conductors, such as a human and a power-cord wire, are separated by a nonconductor, such as air. The capacitor formed in the illustration is made up of the metal of the power lines and the conductive interstitial fluid in the human; the nonconductive air is separating them. The current flows from the power line through the capacitance and into the patient. It then goes out of the left arm into the upper lead of the differential amplifier, and it also goes out of the right arm into the lower lead of the differential amplifier. Usually, the resulting voltages would be the same on both terminals, and they would be common-mode signals. A differential amplifier cancels such signals, and, therefore, the 60-cycle interference does not normally appear on an ECG trace.

However, if the contact resistance of one of the lead surface electrodes is very high because of a poor connection or because the gel has dried out, the AC voltages would not be the same on both terminals. The difference in the resistance in the two leads would result in different levels of AC signal on the differential amplifier terminals. The AC signal would no longer be common-mode and would not be rejected by the amplifier. It would appear instead on the ECG trace as AC interference (noise), as illustrated in Figure 4.10(c). A way to correct AC noise is to check the electrode for sufficient gel or to tighten the electrodes to the skin. Frayed leads or leads that are poorly attached to the ECG panel could also cause the problem.

Standard Lead Connections

The standard lead connections are termed *Lead I, Lead II,* and *Lead III.* The body potentials they carry to the ECG unit are respectively called *I, II,* and *III.* In Figure 4.3(a), the biopotential *I* is the voltage potential drop from the left arm to the right arm due to the electrical activity of the heart. This voltage potential appears at the input terminals of the ECG differential amplifier. The leads are called *bipolar leads* because they are between two points on the body, both of which vary in voltage due to the electrical activity of the heart.

A portion of *I* is fed back to the right leg through a common-mode reduction circuit (CM). This circuit takes a part of the common-mode signal, inverts it by 180 degrees, and applies it to the right leg. This signal tends to cancel the common-mode from the power lines by destructive interference. The destructive interference results because the 180-degree shift in feedback puts the two signals in opposite polarity at all times. Thus, they tend to cancel out each other. This has the effect of reducing any AC interference that might exist.

The output of the ECG amplifier then presents a clean ECG waveform at levels in the order of one volt to the display unit. The display unit is thus enabled to record the trace.

In part (b) of Figure 4.3, lead *II* takes the biopotential *II* produced by the heart as the plus-to-minus voltage drop from the left leg to the right arm and applies it to the ECG differential amplifier. It is then delivered to the display as just described.

Likewise, part (c) of the figure shows how lead *III* connects the voltage *III* to the ECG and delivers it to the display.

Einthoven Triangle

In summary, the three voltages *I, II,* and *III* are measured on the body as:

I—The voltage drop from left arm to right arm.

II—The voltage drop from left leg to right arm.

III—The drop from left leg to left arm.

Anatomically, these points form a triangle on the body, known as the *Einthoven triangle.* As illustrated in Figure 4.4, the voltages may be represented by vectors, having the tail on the negative pole of the potential and the arrowhead on the positive pole of the potential. Thus, in clinical practice, the three voltages are represented as vectors, which are called *frontal-plane vectors* and illustrated in

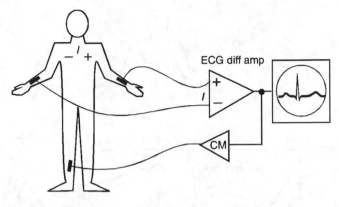

(a) Standard Lead *I*

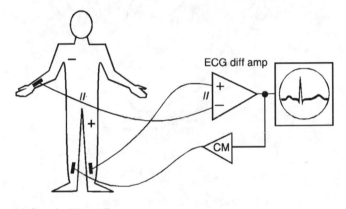

(b) Standard Lead *II*

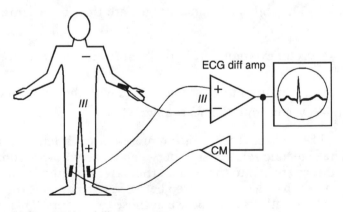

(c) Standard Lead *III*

FIGURE 4.3   Standard lead connections

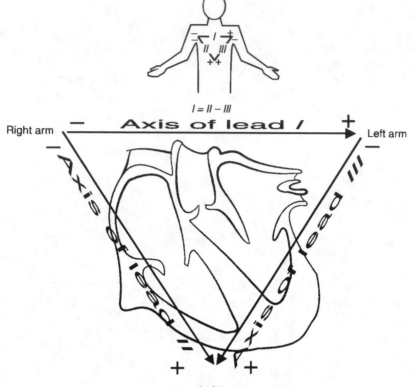

FIGURE 4.4   *Einthoven triangle*

Figure 4.5. The standard lead voltages are then represented as follows:

> *I*—A vector extending from the heart in the horizontal direction (0°).
>
> *II*—A vector from the heart down 60° with the horizontal.
>
> *III*—A vector from the heart down 120°.

More will be said about the vector representation in later sections.

The algebraic relationship between these voltages comes from circuit theory applied to the human thorax. It is a fundamental law of voltage drops that the voltage drop between two points is the same regardless of the path traveled between those two points. This is known as *Kirchhoff's law* of voltages.

That law applied to Figure 4.4 implies that the voltage drop as one travels from the left arm to the right arm equals the drops measured as

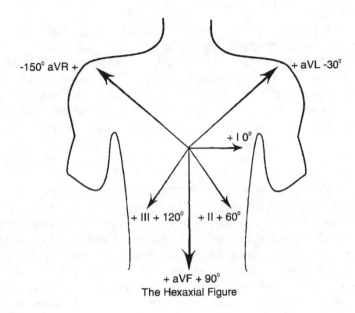

The Hexaxial Figure

FIGURE 4.5   Frontal-plane vectors

one travels from the left arm to the left leg and then to the right arm. In equation form, this implies that

$$I = II - III \qquad (4.1)$$

The minus sign appears because III is a negative drop, in accordance with the polarities assigned in Figure 4.4. The three voltages as arranged on the figure have traditionally been called Einthoven's triangle, in honor of Willem Einthoven, the physiologist and inventor, who studied ECG voltages in 1903.

Equation (4.1) means that only two leads are needed to gather all of the information available to the three leads. This follows from the fact that, using Equation (4.1), the voltage on any one of the leads can be calculated from the other two. In other words, one of the leads is redundant. This is not wasteful, though, because if one of the leads is poorly connected, the information will still be available for diagnosis. This is especially important in ECG units that do diagnosis automatically.

Unipolar Augmented Lead Connections

Another way of gathering the same information about the ECG activity as it appears in the standard leads is through unipolar augmented lead connections. They are called *unipolar leads* because they are measured from one of the limbs to an electrically neutral point. The voltage at the electrically neutral point does not change due to the electrical activity of the heart. These unipolar lead connections are called the augmented right-arm lead (aVR), the augmented left-arm lead (aVL), and the augmented left-foot lead (aVF). The voltage in all of these leads can be calculated from any two of the standard lead voltages. This means that they are all redundant in terms of the information they supply. This raises the question: If they are redundant, why are they measured?

There are several good reasons: (1) as mentioned previously, if one of the leads is poorly connected, the information will still be there; (2) each lead shows the ECG activity from a different perspective, so that the trace from each lead appears different on the display and emphasizes different distinctive features; and (3) historically, a large number of case studies, both formally documented and in the minds of practicing cardiologists using these leads, are available to aid in making diagnosis.

The aVR connection is shown in Figure 4.6(a). The right arm is connected to the positive terminal of the ECG differential amplifier. Two resistors, R, in series are connected from the left arm to the left leg; and the node between the resistors, which is clinically taken to be the electrically neutral point, is connected to the negative terminal of the ECG amplifier. Again, the output of the common-mode reduction circuit is connected to the right leg.

Applying Kirchhoff's law to the voltage drops in the figure yields the relationship

$$aVR = -I - \frac{III}{2} \qquad (4.2)$$

where two resistors form a voltage divider whose output is $III/2$. This equation shows how the aVR can be calculated from the lead I and lead III voltages. The minus sign appears because the polarities of I and III are in the opposite direction from aVR. The III is divided by 2 because the lead III voltage is reduced by the voltage divider resistors, R.

The aVL augmented lead connection is made similarly except the resistors are connected from the right arm and the left leg, as shown in part (b) of Figure 4.6. The node between the resistors is connected to the negative terminal of the ECG amplifier, and the left arm is connected to the positive terminal.

Applying Kirchhoff's law to calculate aVL yields the equation

$$aVL = I - \frac{II}{2} \qquad (4.3)$$

which shows that aVL can be calculated from the lead I and lead II voltages.

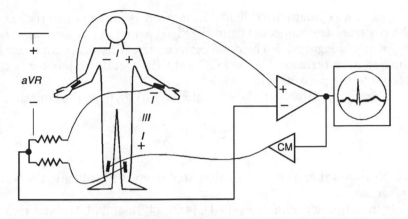

$$aVR = -I - \frac{III}{2}$$ (a)

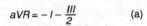

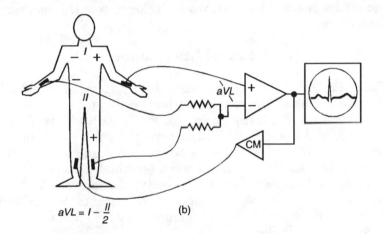

$$aVL = I - \frac{II}{2}$$ (b)

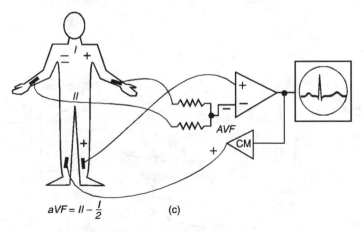

$$aVF = II - \frac{I}{2}$$ (c)

FIGURE 4.6 Unipolar augmented lead connections

The *aVF* augmented lead connection is made similarly except the resistors are connected from the right arm and left arm, as shown in part (c) of Figure 4.6. The node between the resistors is connected to the negative terminal of the ECG amplifier, and the left leg is connected to the positive terminal.

Applying Kirchhoff's law to calculate *aVF* yields the equation

$$aVF = II - \frac{I}{2} \tag{4.4}$$

which shows that *aVF* can be calculated from the lead *I* and the lead *II* voltages.

In summary, Equations (4.1), (4.2), (4.3), and (4.4) show that all of the standard and augmented lead connections can be calculated from any two of the standard lead voltages. That means that four of the six leads are redundant, which helps ensure the accuracy of the display.

Precordial Lead Connections

The chest leads are called *precordial leads*. They are unipolar leads in that they measure the voltage on the chest relative to an electrically neutral point. As illustrated in Figure 4.7, six leads are used to measure one of the precordial lead displays. The three limb leads—right arm—left arm, and left leg—are connected through resistors, *R*, to a single point called the Wilson central terminal. This point is taken as a reference because it stays relatively constant as the ECG trace changes. It is connected to the negative terminal of the ECG amplifier. As usual, the output from the common-mode reduction circuit is connected to the right leg.

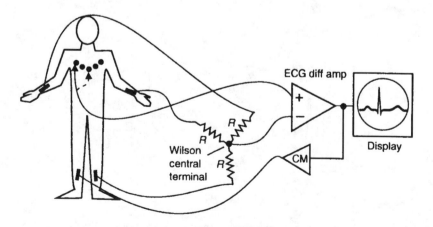

FIGURE 4.7   Precordial lead connections

The precordial lead is connected from one of six anatomical sites on the chest to the positive terminal of the ECG. Because the Wilson central terminal is electrically inactive, essentially all of the electrical changes take place at the precordial lead electrode. It is therefore called a *unipolar* electrode.

The sites of the six possible precordial leads, as illustrated in Figure 4.8(a), are as follows:

V_1—Fourth intercostal space, on the right sternal margin.

V_2—Fourth intercostal space, on the left sternal margin.

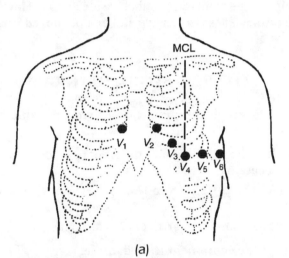

(a)

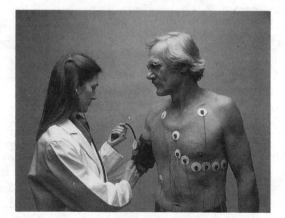

(b)

FIGURE 4.8   (a) The anatomical sites of the six precordial leads (From Kinney et al, p. 80. Used by permission of Mosby). (b) A photograph showing the precordial lead sites (Courtesy of Consolidated Medical Corporation)

V_3—Midway between V_2 and V_4.

V_4—Fifth intercostal space on the midclavicular line (MCL).

V_5—Fifth intercostal space on the anterior axillary line.

V_6—Fifth intercostal space on the midaxillary line.

Because V_1, V_2, and V_3 straddle the heart, they are especially useful in distinguishing what parts of the heart may be abnormal. Because the six sites are relatively closely spaced, it works best to use a small electrode such as a suction cup electrode or a conductive adhesive electrode. The chance of nosocomial infection is reduced somewhat by the use of disposable conductive adhesive electrodes. However, the suction cup electrode is less expensive and can be moved from site to site conveniently.

THE ECG BLOCK DIAGRAM

The electrocardiograph equipment is designed to achieve the following goals:

- To amplify the ECG signal and prepare it for display or further signal processing.
- To protect the patient from leakage current and other electrical hazards.
- To minimize noise and artifacts in the signal.
- To protect the equipment from damage.

A block diagram that achieves these goals is shown in Figure 4.9. Ten patient cables are attached to surface electrodes on the body. ECG signals from the body are applied first to a *defibrillator protection circuit*. This prevents a blowout of the ECG circuits, which may occur if the patient is defibrillated. The defibrillator pulse can be several thousand volts, and needs to be shunted away from the ECG unit electronics. The defibrillator protection circuit does this task.

The ECG signals then pass into a *buffer*, or a high-input impedance circuit. The input resistance, approximately 5 megohms, is more than ten times the skin–electrode resistance of a normally connected patient lead. The skin–electrode resistance is therefore negligible and does not introduce any significant imbalances into the unit. This high resistance isolates the patient from the electronics of the equipment, and keeps leakage currents to low, safe levels.

Next, the signal is selected by the *lead selector* switch, which has up to 12 positions to make the connections of Lead *I*, Lead *II*, Lead *III*, *aVR*, *aVL*, *aVF*, and V_1 through V_6. The signal selected is applied to the differential amplifier.

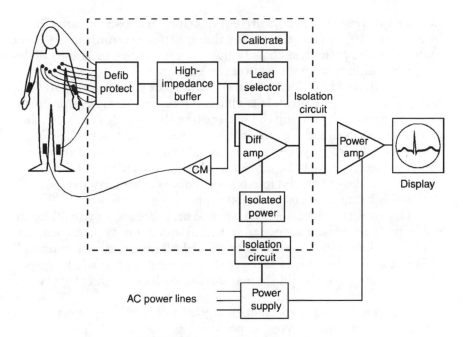

FIGURE 4.9   An ECG block diagram

The output of the buffer is also processed by the *common-mode reduction circuit* (CM) and fed back to the right leg to reduce 60-cycle noise in the ECG.

The output of the differential amplifier is passed through an *isolation circuit* into a *power amplifier* that, in turn, drives the display unit for the ECG trace.

To run the electronics, a *power supply* is necessary (Figure 4.9). The voltage in the 110 V AC power line is reduced below 20 V DC by the power supply in order to run the electronics. To isolate the patient from leakage currents associated with the AC power line, an isolation circuit is employed. In that way, the lead leakage current is kept below 10 microamp, and chances of the 110 V AC shorting to the patient leads are extremely remote.

Artifacts in the ECG

Besides the two artifacts discussed previously—baseline wander and 60-cycle hum—other signals on the ECG trace that do not originate from the heart may be caused by skeletal muscle contraction or tremor, dirty or loose electrodes, pacemaker artifacts, radiation pickup from an electrosurgical unit (ESU) or another radio frequency source, magnet resonator imager (MRI) interference, baseline wander due to respiratory movement, lead reversal or misconnection, or loose or faulty leads (see Figure 4.10). In fact, almost any therapeutic, electronic instrument attached to the patient, such as IV pumps, ventilators, or kidney dialysis units, can induce an artifact on the ECG trace.

The effects of muscle tremor, shown in part (c) of Figure 4.10, look much like a 60-cycle hum. It is characterized by being less uniform. One can check it by having the patient flex the muscles near the electrodes and observing the changes. Due to nervous tension, the patient may not be able to relax enough to get rid of all the noise. If this is the case, the electrodes may be moved to another site closer to bone, as on the wrist or above the clavicle bones. This is especially necessary if the ECG is being taken on an ambulatory patient.

Dry or dirty electrodes can cause an increase in the 60-cycle noise by introducing impedance imbalances. Or skin movement under the electrode may introduce irregularities, as shown in part (d) of Figure 4.10. The remedy is to replace the electrode or add some gel, clean the site with a mild soap-and-water solution, and reapply the electrode.

Interference from an electrosurgical unit (ESU) in the room is caused by strong radio waves, as powerful as those from a small broadcast band radio transmitter. This interference may completely distort the trace so that it is unrecognizable. Changing the position of the ESU cables or the ECG cables may cut the coupling and reduce the interference. Fortunately, the ESU is only used intermittently, so a reading can be taken when the machine is off. Many ECGs are designed to suppress ESU radiation. This is relatively easy to do because, being at approximately 500 kHz, the ESU is widely separated in frequency from the ECG.

MRI interference introduces into the environment a strong magnetic field that may pull the trace toward the MRI unit and distort its morphology.

Other errors in application can result from misconnections. The leads are sometimes color coded to help reduce their being put at the wrong body site. However, it is best if the attendant follows the leads from the instrumentation input to the appropriate site on the patient in accordance with the Figures 4.3 to 4.7 in this chapter. Because there is no standard, the color coding depends on the manufacturer of the ECG unit. In practice, someone might substitute the wrong color lead because it is available and can be made to work. This could cause confusion. The color code does not help when all six precordial leads are connected simultaneously; therefore, careful checking is necessary.

A reversal of the leads, shown in part (e) of Figure 4.10, can cause severe distortion in the ECG. If, for example, the patient cables for the left arm and the right arm were reversed, the Lead *I* display would be reversed, and Leads *II* and *III* would be distorted. If not recognized in time, this could lead to a confusion in interpretation.

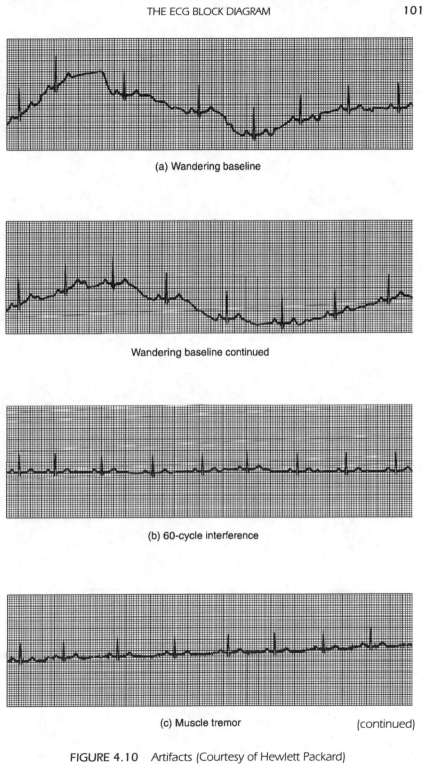

(a) Wandering baseline

Wandering baseline continued

(b) 60-cycle interference

(c) Muscle tremor   (continued)

FIGURE 4.10   Artifacts (Courtesy of Hewlett Packard)

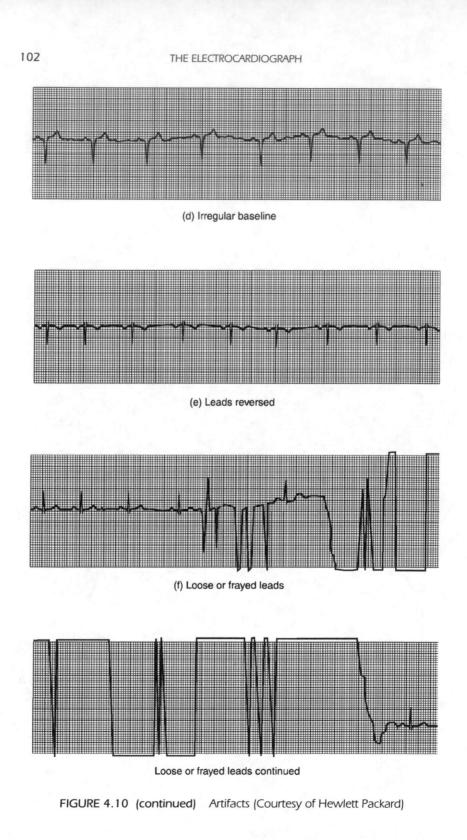

(d) Irregular baseline

(e) Leads reversed

(f) Loose or frayed leads

Loose or frayed leads continued

FIGURE 4.10 (continued)   Artifacts (Courtesy of Hewlett Packard)

If the leads are loose, either due to dried electrodes, deteriorated adhesive, or a poor connection, the trace may move violently across the screen with the slightest movement from the patient or disturbance of the leads. A frayed or loose electrical connection at the front panel could cause the same artifact. Such traces are shown in part (f) of Figure 4.10. The remedy is to reprepare the electrodes or replace the cables.

Normal ECG Traces

The normal ECG traces of the 12-lead system are given in Figure 4.11 as used by the U.S. Navy. Each small division on the horizontal scale represents 40 ms, and each vertical division is 0.1 mV. The speed of the trace is 25 millimeters per second. The most distinctive feature in all cases is the *QRS* complex. The *T* wave is the next largest, and the *P* wave is the smallest and sometimes difficult to detect.

The standard limb leads, *I, II, III,* and the augmented leads, *aVR, aVF,* and *aVL* measure the voltages on the frontal plane of the body. These form vectors in the superior, inferior, right, and left directions. The precordial leads measure cardiac voltages, forming vectors in the anterior, posterior, right, and left directions. Further discussion of these vectors appears in Chapter 5. Routine monitoring is often done with lead *II* because it has a strong *QRS* complex and the *P* wave and *T* wave are quite distinct. For long-term monitoring, other leads may be prescribed. For example, the precordial lead V_1 may be prescribed because it gives the most valuable information about arrhythmias.

Alarmed ECG Traces

Modern 12-lead ECGs go beyond the measurement and monitoring task and attempt diagnosis. Computer processing of ECGs does very detailed ECG-based diagnosis of heart disease. Smaller units may respond to changes in the ECG that require immediate nursing attention. These include bradycardia and tachycardia or emergency situations such as paroxysmal (sudden) ventricular tachycardia, premature ventricular contractions (PVCs), asystole (lack of ventricular contraction), or ventricular fibrillation (VF) (see Figure 4.12).

ECG traces of normal sinus rhythm, sinus bradycardia and sinus tachycardia are compared in parts (a) to (c) of Figure 4.12. The lower limit of the bpm alarm may be set anywhere from 40 to 60 bpm, depending upon what is judged to be normal for the patient. Likewise, the tachycardia trace usually has the alarm set above 100 bpm.

Paroxysmal ventricular tachycardia (VT), illustrated in part (e), occurs at heart rates above 150 bpm. It comes on suddenly and may

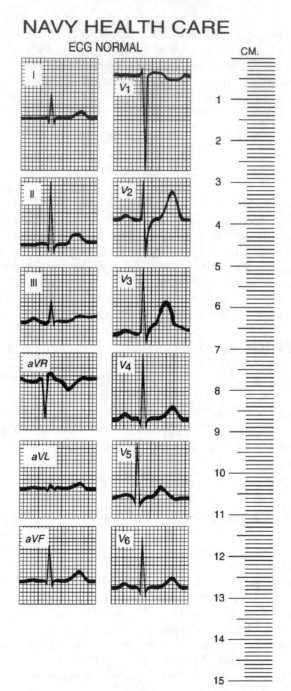

FIGURE 4.11   Normal ECG traces

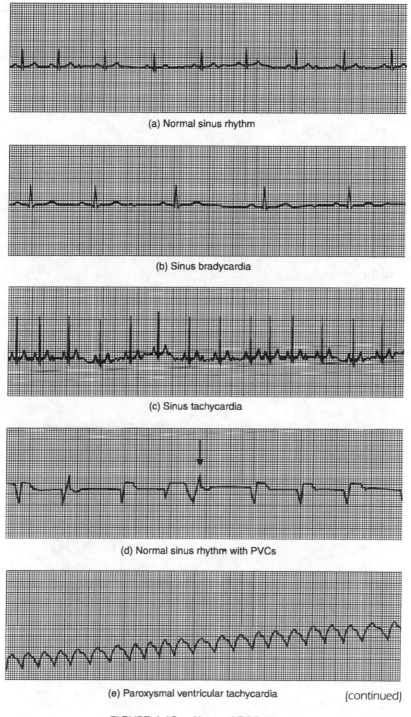

(a) Normal sinus rhythm

(b) Sinus bradycardia

(c) Sinus tachycardia

(d) Normal sinus rhythm with PVCs

(e) Paroxysmal ventricular tachycardia   (continued)

FIGURE 4.12   Alarmed ECG traces

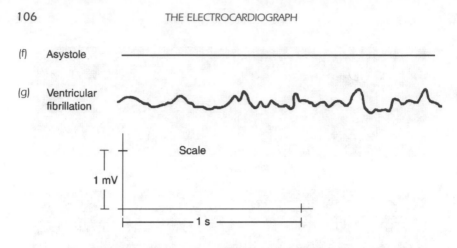

FIGURE 4.12 (continued)   Alarmed ECG traces

deteriorate to a ventricular fibrillation. It is therefore life threatening and requires emergency treatment.

Frequent PVCs are illustrated in part (d) of the figure. They may originate in the right or left ventricle, and they may be unifocal or multifocal. If the clinical setting is of acute myocardial infarction, they are considered dangerous and aggressive treatment may be necessary. However, as with any arrhythmia, the rule is to treat the patient, not the monitor. That is, the decision to give treatment must be made by a qualified health-care provider.

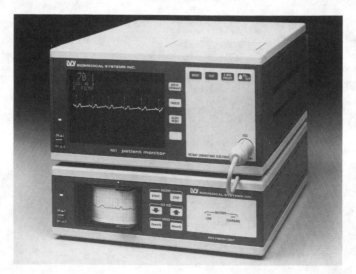

FIGURE 4.13   An ECG unit that may be battery operated (Courtesy of IVY Biomedical Systems, Inc.)

All of these situations can initiate a monitoring alarm. Because the *QRS* complex is the largest feature of the ECG trace, a threshold detector that passes only the part of the wave that exceeds the threshold provides pulses that could be counted to yield the bpms. It requires only two beats to make the measurement and, therefore, could detect a PVC.

Asystole appears as a flat trace, as shown in Figure 4.12 (f), and may be alarmed. VF has no *QRS* complex, but the fibrillation contains frequency components above 150 cycles per second. The simultaneous absence of the *QRS* and the presence of signals above 150 cycles per second could trigger an alarm for VF.

An ECG monitor is shown in Figure 4.13. A trace is shown on the cathode-ray tube (video display), and the same trace is also shown on the paper chart below. This unit may be battery operated.

REFERENCES

Conover, M. B. *Pocket Nurse Guide to Electrocardiography.* St. Louis: C.V. Mosby Co., 1986.

Hewlett Packard Staff. *ECG Techniques: Applications Manual* 5952–3366. Waltham, MA: Hewlett Packard Company, 1972.

Kinney, Packa, Andreoli, Zipes. *Comprehensive Cardiac Care.* 7th ed. St. Louis: C. V. Mosby, 1991.

Walraven, Gail. *Basic Arrhythmias.* 2nd ed. Englewood Cliffs, N.J.: Prentice-Hall, Inc., 1986.

EXERCISES

1. Draw an equivalent circuit of the lead *I* ECG showing how the information flows from the heart to the display.

2. What factors affect the polarization potential?

3. What is the effect of the polarization voltage on the display?

4. What causes baseline wander in an ECG display?

5. What action should be taken to correct baseline wander?

6. What is the source of 60-cycle interference in an ECG trace?

7. Name three factors related to the patient leads that could cause 60-cycle interference in an ECG trace.

8. Why does a poor skin–electrode connection cause 60-cycle interference on an ECG trace?

9. State Kirchhoff's law.

10. What formula relates the surface potentials associated with leads *I*, *II*, and *III*?

11. What is meant by the statement that some of the leads on an ECG are redundant?

12. Among the three standard leads and the three augmented leads, how many are redundant?

13. Why are redundant leads used in the ECG measurement?

14. Draw the circuit diagram for the aVR lead connection.

15. Draw the circuit diagram for the aVF lead connection.

16. Using the circuit diagram in exercise 15, derive the formula that can be used to compute aVF from the lead I and lead II ECGs.

17. Draw the circuit diagram for one of the precordial lead connections.

18. List the anatomical sites for placement of the ECG precordial leads.

19. What are the design goals for an ECG unit?

20. Why is high-voltage protection to the front end of an ECG unit necessary?

21. What is the function of the high-impedance buffer in an ECG?

22. Name the 12 lead positions.

23. Other than baseline wander and 60-cycle hum, list the causes of artifacts on an ECG display.

24. What action should be taken to reduce artifacts due to skeletal muscle interference?

25. What action should be taken to eliminate 60-cycle hum?

26. Describe the characteristics of MRI interference in an ECG display.

27. Describe distortion due to strong ESU radiation.

28. Why is a color scheme for the patient leads limited in use?

29. Why are the chest leads more difficult to attach?

30. Why is the V_1 lead often preferred for long-term monitoring?

31. Name five commonly alarmed heart conditions that are easily recognized on ECG traces.

32. What distinguishes a VF trace?

33. Name one possible precursor of VF.

CHAPTER 5

Microprocessor-Based Equipment

THE MICROPROCESSOR

The microprocessor is a computer fabricated entirely on a thin wafer of silicon crystal only one or two square inches in area. The chip only costs about ten dollars. Because it is so small, inexpensive, and complex, it has had a profound impact on machine development since its invention in the 1970s. Relevant to this discussion is its impact on medical instrumentation. In fact, most of the patient care instrumentation discussed in this book, including defibrillators, pacemakers, IV pumps, ventilators, and ECG monitors, has been greatly improved by the use of the microprocessor.

Because the microprocessor is a computer, it can perform a logical analysis of the data fed to it. That is, it can accept raw physiological data, such as ECG patterns, and analyze them. From this analysis, the microprocessor can illuminate a display identifying disease or giving the health-care provider diagnostic options. In some cases, diagnostic data not available to a human observer are detected by the microprocessor, which then delivers lifesaving therapy without human intervention. This is done specifically in the case of the automatic implantable cardiac defibrillator (AICD), which will be described in Chapter 6.

One of the best examples of a microprocessor is a hand calculator, which consists of an input unit (the keyboard), a display, and a microprocessor chip. For just a few dollars, an undergraduate can use it to do almost all of the calculating in the curriculum, including sophisticated mathematics. It is also powered by a battery that lasts for years. This is probably the most efficient and elegant machine ever devised. It is its calculating power and low cost that make it so important to medical instrumentation.

Anatomy of a Microprocessor

The electronics of a microprocessor can be constructed of arrangements of microscopic etchings called *pn junctions*. To construct these junctions, a wafer of silicon is treated first with a gas such as arsenic followed by a gas such as aluminum vapor. A photographic developing process is then used to etch out millions of these junctions and connect them into electronic circuits. The process uses such inexpensive materials and is so automated that each wafer, which consists of millions of parts, can be stamped out for only a few dollars.

All of the circuits in a microprocessor can be constructed from three basic logical units: an AND gate, an OR gate, and a NOT gate. Not only are these concepts essential to the description of a microprocessor but to other medical instruments as well.

> *AND gate*—An electronic circuit that gives an output on terminal C only when both inputs A *and* B receive a stimulus. Its symbol follows:

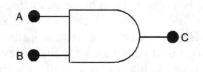

> *OR gate*—An electronic circuit that gives an output stimulus at C when terminals A or B *or* both A and B are stimulated. Its symbol follows:

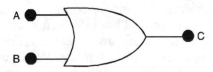

> *NOT gate*—An electronic circuit that inhibits an input stimulus applied to terminal A from appearing at terminal C, but presents an output when the stimulus is zero.

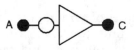

All of the mathematical operations and logical decisions a computer makes are sequences of these logical functions. A microprocessor in medical equipment uses this logic to make calculations on physiological data and to make if/then clause decisions.

Machine Language

Human language consists of about 30 sounds, which make up speech. Written language uses almost the same number of symbols, namely, the 26 letters of the alphabet. Machine language consists of only two symbols: 1 and 0. Strings of these two symbols are called *binary numbers*.

The 1 may represent the presence of a stimulus, and the 0 may represent the absence of a stimulus. Such stimuli in the human body are quantities like pressure or flow. The stimulus in the machine usually consists of a voltage.

The correlation between written language and machine language is a standard code such that each letter of the alphabet and each number from zero to nine is represented as a binary number, or machine word, with a string of 1s and 0s. For example:

ALPHA NUMERIC SYMBOL	MACHINE WORD
A	1000001
B	1000010
C	1000011
⋮	⋮
1	0110001
2	0110010
3	0110011
⋮	⋮

This table is extended to include all of the symbols normally seen on the computer keyboard, and is called the ASCII (pronounced "ask key") code. The microprocessor manipulates these machine words to do the logical operations necessary to process physiological data and make decisions.

Microprocessor Block Diagram

Physiological data appears in the body as a continuous and smooth function of time, called an *analog* signal. To be processed in a microprocessor, it must be converted into a *digital* signal. This may be done by sampling the value of the signal at fixed time intervals and recording the signal as that value until the next sample is taken. The number is rounded to one of a set number of values, consistent with the desired accuracy of measurement.

For any particular sampling period, the digital signal value is represented as a binary word and applied to the input of the microprocessor, as illustrated in Figure 5.1. The components of a microprocessor illustrated in the figure are described as follows:

CPU—The computer processing unit. The region on the chip where all of the mathematical and logical data manipulation is done.

Bus—Connecting pathways in cables of 8 to 32 wires, which conduct signals around the microprocessor.

Memory—The region on the chip were digital words may be stored. Each memory location consists of 8 to 32 points on the chip, each about the size of a living cell. To address the memory, one activates a set of gates so that those points are connected to the *data bus*, those wires dedicated to passing data. One of two values of voltage at those points determines whether a 1 or a 0 of the binary word is stored. That voltage will retain its given value unless it is changed by a signal on the data bus.

Address bus—Those wires that connect the signal from the CPU to the memory and activate a pathway from the data bus to the memory location addressed. This enables the signal in memory to flow along the data bus either to the CPU or to the output unit, or it may connect the input unit to that memory location.

Control bus—Those wires that send timing signals from the CPU to the input unit, the output unit, and the memory chip.

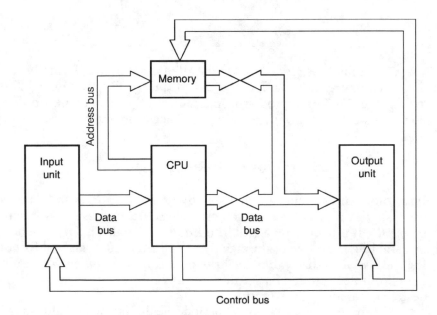

FIGURE 5.1   A microprocessor block diagram

Capabilities of the Microprocessor

Because the signal is represented as binary numbers in a microprocessor, the microprocessor can perform all standard mathematical operations, such as addition, subtraction, multiplication, and division; it can also be programmed to do calculus on those signals. The microprocessor can compare these signals with a data base in memory and make comparative decisions. It does this by means of a computer program stored in the memory and activated by the CPU. If properly programmed, the microprocessor can do all of the functions of a desktop computer. The output unit of the microprocessor will either deliver a signal back to the physiological system, such as for therapy, or drive an output display with information for the human observer.

APPLICATIONS

Over the past decade, the microprocessor has become an integral part of several important pieces of patient-care equipment. It is used to control ventilators that assist patients in breathing. It is used in pacemakers to make them more responsive to human needs and more readily programmable. It is used in IV pumps as well. Specific ways the microprocessor improves these devices is discussed in the chapters on those topics. The idea of a computer so small and inexpensive that each machine can have its own dedicated computer, which can even be implanted in the body, is revolutionary; and it is the reason why a systematic discussion of the device for health-care providers is given here.

The microprocessor has also been important in the area of diagnostic equipment. A computer tomography (CT) scanner would not be possible without a dedicated computer. Without it, the image calculation by hand would take weeks, whereas it takes seconds in the machine. The same could be said for the magnetic resonance imager (MRI). The effectiveness of other imaging devices, such as the conventional X ray and ultrasonic machines, has also been greatly enhanced by computer image processing.

In patient-monitoring equipment, microprocessor-based signal processing has made the measuring of parameters more accurate and faster than can be done by hand. Here the example of ECG signal analysis is illustrated.

Microprocessor-Based ECG Analysis

The features of the microprocessor that make it seem almost like an extension of the human mind are its ability to do logical analysis, its memory, and its ability to learn complex procedures. The learning is done when someone loads a program. In fact, this frees people from having to learn the complex procedures themselves. The microprocessor does them faster and more accurately.

In order for a microprocessor to analyze an ECG waveform, it must first be placed in its memory. To put it in memory, the voltage value of the ECG waveform is measured at fixed intervals of approximately one millisecond. Each successive value is stored in a different memory location until one cycle of waveform is inserted.

Once it is stored, the microprocessor program can call it up at the same time rate. Likewise, many cycles of the ECG waveform can be stored in memory, each successive value being represented by a binary number.

With that information in memory, the program can call forth the data to measure clinically significant features, such as the duration and magnitude of the P wave, the R wave, the S–T segment, and the T wave (Figure 3.16). It also may measure the duration of the P–R interval, the P–R segment, the QRS complex, and the S–T interval. These measurements can be made from 12 different ECG lead connections.

Also, from the information in the memory, one can measure the R–R interval between successive beats. Comparisons can be made with normal values based on either the general population or the patient's own ECG waveform.

With the advent of the microprocessor, the clinician no longer has to make calculations from ECG waveforms. The machine does it faster and more accurately. This is a convenience and possible cost savings, but it is not always absolutely necessary. However, there are certain functions the microprocessor can perform that are almost impossible for humans unaided by the machine to do.

One such task is monitoring a patient for intermittent irregularities, such as premature ventricular contractions (PVCs), premature atrial contraction (PAC), paroxysmal atrial tachycardia (PAT), paroxysmal ventricular tachycardia (PVT), ventricular fibrillation (VF), or asystole. All of these conditions occur suddenly and unexpectedly. Human monitoring would require that one watch the ECG display constantly. No one can accurately do such a boring task for a long time. In searching for PVCs, one needs to find as few as 30 per hour to diagnose a pathological condition. The machine can do such observation as long as required, at a fraction of the cost of a human observer.

Ambulatory Monitoring

The microprocessor is used in portable ECG units called *Holter monitors*, which can be worn by ambulatory cardiac patients so that intermittent arrhythmias can be studied. The patient wears an ECG monitor about the size of a portable radio and is free to move about within the hospital or at home. When arrhythmias are detected, the associated ECG waveform is stored in the microprocessor memory. At set periods, usually from 24 to 48 hours, a printout discloses complete arrhythmia information. These monitors may be programmed with the patient's normal ECG data to give a basis for arrhythmia detection. Information about deviations in the voltage level of the S–T segment are also available. Normally, this is zero, but higher or lower values relate to possible cardiac ischemia.

Because the program directs the observer only to the abnormal portions of the ECG, which are stored in memory, these can be conveniently scanned several times for more accurate observation.

Vector Cardiography

Vector cardiography involves many calculations that are much better done by the microprocessor than by hand. The heart vector is made up of a voltage between the surface of a sphere and the center of the heart. The vector is defined not only by its voltage value but also its direction. This is an idealized concept that has been adopted by convention and does not have a precise biophysical basis. However, the vector is useful in indicating the location of infarcted tissue in diseased hearts.

The heart vector is made up, by convention, of the sum of three components as follows:

V_6—A vector directed horizontally in the frontal plane from the subject's right to left. Its value at any point in time is the voltage of the V_6 lead of the ECG.

aVF—A vector directed vertically from the superior to inferior direction. Its value at any point in time is the voltage of the aVF lead.

V_2—A vector directed horizontally in the transverse plane from posterior to anterior. Its value is the voltage of the V_2 lead.

These three vectors and the resultant heart vector are illustrated in Figure 5.2. Here, the vector is illustrated as it appears at the peak of the R wave, normally occurring 0.04 seconds after the onset of the QRS complex. This vector is important because in a cardiac patient, it is usually directed away from the infarcted area and aids in its location.

The component of the heart vector lying in each of the three planes can be presented individually. For example, the path of the vectors in the frontal plane, derived from the aVF and V_6 leads, is shown in Figure 5.3. At each point in time, the vector makes an angle

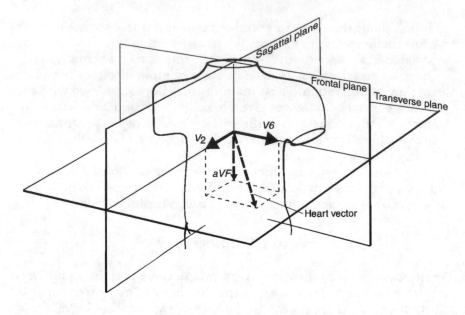

FIGURE 5.2   The heart vector

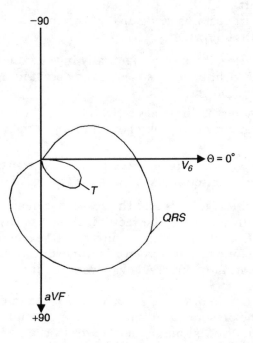

FIGURE 5.3   An ECG presented on the frontal plane

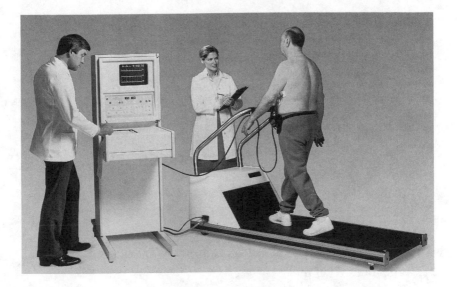

FIGURE 5.4 An ECG stress test. The patient exercises on the treadmill to induce stress. (Courtesy of Quinton Instrument Company)

θ with the horizontal axis. The *P* wave sweeps out the smallest loop first. It normally lies between the angles from 0 to 75 degrees. The larger *QRS* trace normally lies between –30 and 90 degrees. The *T* wave illustrated in Figure 5.3 normally lies between –30 and 60 degrees. A discussion of some pathologies that are reflected in the abnormalities of these vector patterns is discussed by R. Plonsey (see the References). A patient being monitored for ECG under stress is shown in Figure 5.4.

REFERENCES

Mark, R. G., and G. B. Moody. "Arrhythmia Analysis, Automated." *Encyclopedia of Medical Devices and Instrumentation.* vol 1 Edited by J. G. Webster. New York: John Wiley & Sons, 1988: 195–225.

Plonsey, R. "Electrocardiography." *Encyclopedia of Medical Devices and Instrumentation.* vol 2 Edited by J. G. Webster. New York: John Wiley & Sons, 1988: 1017–40.

Thakor, N. V. "Electrocardiographic Monitors." *Encyclopedia of Medical Devices and Instrumentation.* vol 2 Edited by J. G. Webster. New York: John Wiley & Sons, 1988: 1002–17.

Thakor, N. V. "Computers in Electrocardiography." *Encyclopedia of Medical Devices and Instrumentation.* vol 2 Edited by J. G. Webster. New York: John Wiley & Sons, 1988: 1040–61.

EXERCISES

1. Describe a microprocessor.
2. Name four medical instruments improved by the microprocessor.
3. What is the basic building block of a microprocessor?
4. What is the approximate cost of a microprocessor chip?
5. From what logical units can a microprocessor be constructed?
6. What is an electronic logical circuit that gives an output only when both inputs receive a simulus?
7. Draw the symbols of an AND and an OR gate.
8. Define a NOT gate.
9. What are binary numbers?
10. What function does the ASCII code serve?
11. What does CPU mean?
12. Describe a bus used in a microprocessor.
13. This region on a chip consists of 32 points, each about the size of a living cell, from which binary numbers can be retrieved. What is it?
14. In what part of a μP chip is data processed?
15. Besides being able to do arithmetic operations, what can the μP do?
16. Why is a dedicated computer necessary to get a CT image?

CHAPTER 6

The Defibrillator and CPR

The *defibrillator* is an electrical device that delivers a pulse of therapeutic current intended to reverse a ventricular fibrillation (VF) or a life-threatening ventricular tachycardia (VT) in the heart of a patient. As was mentioned in Chapter 1, a current applied to the surface of the body in excess of 80 milliamps and less than 1 ampere such that it passes through the heart is apt to cause it to fibrillate. The result is that the cardiac output falls to less than that required to sustain life. This is electrocution. However, if the current exceeds 1 ampere, it carries enough energy to cause all of the cardiac muscle fibers to contract simultaneously and cause the heart to stop fibrillating.

The current pulse needs to be controlled very carefully. If it is too small, it causes fibrillation, and if it is too large, it can cause burn injuries.

DEFIBRILLATOR PRINCIPLES

The early clinical applications of defibrillation in 1956 by P. M. Zoll used an AC current pulse to defibrillate with some success. However, the reliability was significantly improved in 1962 when B. Lown introduced a defibrillator that delivered a short DC pulse of current to the heart through the chest wall. Defibrillation occurs because the strong current stimulus causes simultaneous contraction of all of the muscles in the heart. The first region to repolarize after the pulse is the sinoatrial (SA) node. It, therefore, regains control of the pacing of the heart.

The effective and safe use of the defibrillator depends upon the proper diagnosis of the symptoms of sudden cardiac death (SCD) and upon quick response. Accurate diagnosis is crucial because the defibrillator pulse can induce fibrillation into a heart that is normally beating. The need for quick response is necessary because the probability of reversing a fibrillation with a defibrillator declines rapidly after only one minute. Therefore, the effectiveness of the defibrillator has been improved by making self-diagnostic models available, especially to people with less medical training, such as fire fighters, paramedical professionals, and even laypeople in the home of a cardiac patient. These people decrease the response time by their close availability to the victim of SCD who inherently has little or no warning. In addition, implanted defibrillators are available to patients who have survived SCD and are susceptible to further attacks.

Lown Defibrillator Circuit

An electrical circuit introduced by Lown to deliver a short, high-current pulse to a patient is shown in Figure 6.1. To prepare the defibrillator for external use, it is necessary to charge the capacitor up to between 1,000 and 6,000 volts. This is done by putting the switch in the charge position, so that the battery voltage, stepped up to these high levels, can be applied to the capacitor. The capacitor consists of two pieces of metal separated by an insulating material. If it is made to stand alone, the capacitor will hold its charge for a long time, minutes or even hours in some cases. That is, the capacitor stores energy, W_A, which develops a voltage, V, across its metal plates. The amount of energy in units of joules is given by

$$W_A = C \frac{V^2}{2} \tag{6.1}$$

where C is the value of the capacitance measured in units of farads and V is the voltage across the capacitor. In other words, the energy stored in the capacitor is proportional to the square of the voltage between its plates. The amount of energy typically stored in the capacitor

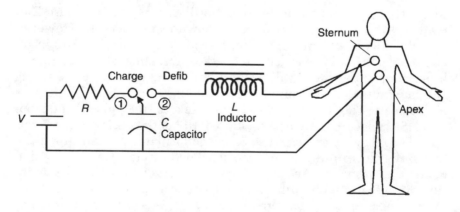

FIGURE 6.1   The Lown Defibrillator Circuit

of a defibrillator, so that it can be later delivered to the patient, ranges from 50 to 400 joules.

Defibrillator Pulse Voltage and Energy

It is important for the defibrillator user to understand the voltage pulse output because its shape is an indicator of proper defibrillator operation. Early defibrillators had an erroneous waveform and were not reliable. An understanding of how the energy is distributed among the human–machine interface components determines whether the patient receives the appropriate therapy or whether an injury is inflicted.

The defibrillator pulse is generated by the basic circuit as shown in Figure 6.1. After the capacitor has been charged with the switch in position 1, the defibrillator is ready to deliver a voltage pulse to the patient. This delivery is made by putting the switch in the discharge position, 2. A voltage waveform across the patient is developed in the shape shown in Figure 6.2. The current is zero at the instant after the

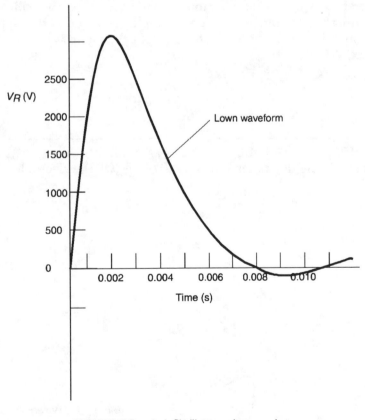

FIGURE 6.2   A defibrillator voltage pulse

switch is thrown because the energy goes into building up a magnetic field around the inductor, L. As that magnetic field builds up, the current, and therefore the voltage, increases in the paddle and patient resistances, causing the initial rise in voltage in the waveform. After the energy stored in the capacitor becomes depleted, the current falls, causing the waveform to peak and then diminish to zero again. The oscillation of the energy between the capacitor and inductor after the initial pulse sometimes causes a small ripple to follow, but that should have no significant physiological effect. The inductor and capacitor values are chosen to make a pulse—in Figure 6.2, for example, to peak at about 2,600 volts and have a duration of approximately 7 milliseconds.

The total energy available from the capacitor is calculated from Equation (6.1). All of this energy does not get into the patient. Some is lost in the internal resistance of the defibrillator circuit, R_D, and some is wasted in the paddle–skin resistance, R_E. To calculate how much of this energy gets to the patient resistance, R_T, consider the equivalent circuit in Figure 6.3. The four resistors in this circuit are in series. Therefore, the current in each of them is the same. And the energy absorbed by any one resistor is proportional to the total available energy, according to the voltage division principle discussed in the Appendix, Section A.1. For example, the formula for the energy absorbed by the thorax, W_T, is

$$W_T = \frac{R_T}{R_T + 2R_E + R_D} W_A \tag{6.2}$$

EXAMPLE 6.1 A defibrillator has an available energy, W_A, of 200 joules (J). If the thorax resistance is 40 ohms (Ω), the electrode–skin re-

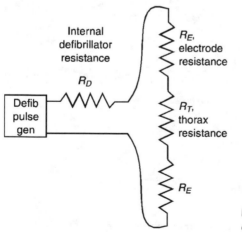

FIGURE 6.3 Equivalent circuit of the defibrillator–patient interface

sistance of a paddle with sufficient electrode gel is 30 ohms and the internal resistance of the defibrillator is 10 ohms. Calculate the energy delivered to the thorax of the patient.

Solution In this case, R_T = 40 ohms, R_E = 30 ohms, and R_D = 10 ohms. So Equation (6.2) yields

$$W_T = \frac{40 \ \Omega}{40 \ \Omega + 2 \ (30 \ \Omega) + 10 \ \Omega} \times 200 = 72.7 \text{ J}$$

This calculation shows that less than half of the available energy gets into the patient where it can defibrillate the heart. Most of the energy is absorbed in the paddles where it is dissipated as heat in the paddle and the skin.

EXAMPLE 6.2 The defibrillator has an available energy of 200 J. The thorax resistance is 40 ohms. The paddles are not properly covered with gel, so each paddle has an electrode–skin resistance of 200 ohms. Calculate how much of the available energy gets into the thorax of the patient.

Solution Here, R_T = 40 ohms, R_D = 10 ohms, and R_E = 200 ohms. So Equation (6.2) yields

$$W_A = \frac{40 \ \Omega}{40 \ \Omega + 2(200 \ \Omega) + 10 \ \Omega} \times 200 = 17.8 \text{ J}$$

In this case, only 17.8 joules of energy get into the thorax of the patient. This probably would not be enough energy to defibrillate a heart. Furthermore, because most of the circuit resistance is in the paddle–skin interface, most of the energy would be dissipated there (in this case, 182 joules). That energy in the paddle–skin interface would be converted to heat and could cause a skin burn. Thus, in this case, the consequence of not putting the proper amount of gel on the paddle is that the heart will not defibrillate and the skin will be burned. Even if the energy setting was turned up to achieve a defibrillation of the heart, it could cost the patient an unnecessary skin burn.

Paddle sizes range from 8 to 13 cm in diameter for adults (4.5 cm for infants). When the skin is properly gelled and a firm pressure is applied, the transthoracic ranges from 27 to 170 ohms. (See Crockett, p. 25.)

Diagnostic Defibrillator

Ventricular fibrillation is a common initial rhythm in sudden cardiac death. Early defibrillation is accepted as the most effective means of improving survival rates in ventricular fibrillation. The greatest impediment to early defibrillation is the fact that many cardiac arrests occur outside the hospital. When communities added early prehospital defibrillation to their Advanced Cardiac Life Support (ACLS) protocols, survival rates improved. Unfortunately, one of the major hazards in using a defibrillator is the misdiagnosis of a fibrillating heart. The major symptoms visible without the aid of diagnostic equipment are a loss of consciousness, dilated pupils, lack of pulse, and apnea. These symptoms require skill and training to assess and can be misinterpreted. If the defibrillating current is delivered to a normal heart, and if it hits during the T wave (when the heart is most vulnerable), it may cause the heart to fibrillate. Therefore, it is necessary to have positive evidence that the heart is fibrillating before the defibrillator is used. This may be obtained from the ECG waveform, as illustrated in Figure 6.4. The fibrillating ECG is characterized by a lack of QRS complexes and a visible component of approximately 150-cycle oscillations.

In an attempt to provide early defibrillation to more of the population, a large number of emergency service people, such as firemen and policemen, who are not used to treating arrhythmias have been trained in the use of the simple automatic external or diagnostic defibrillator, which is illustrated in the block diagram of Figure 6.5. The operation of this defibrillator is best explained by beginning with the patient who is wired with four ECG leads placed in the standard position. The ECG waveform information is processed by the ECG unit to the lower left. The output waveform is then applied to the QRS detector and the fibrillation detector. If the QRS is present, a signal will be applied to the upper lead of the upper AND gate. Then if the attendant pushes the defib switch, placing a signal on the lower lead also, the AND gate will deliver an inhibiting signal to the defibrillator pulse generator. (An AND gate generates an output signal only when stimulus is present on both the upper *and* the lower input terminals.) Thus, an unnecessary defibrillating pulse is kept from the patient.

If, on the other hand, there is no QRS and the fibrillation detector delivers a stimulating pulse to the lower lead of the lower AND gate, then when the attendant activates the defib switch, a stimulus will be put on both terminals of that gate, and its output will trigger the defibrillator. Thus, the defibrillator will deliver a therapeutic current pulse through the large electrodes on the sternum and apex to the patient's chest. An automatic advisory defibrillator is shown in Figure 6.6.

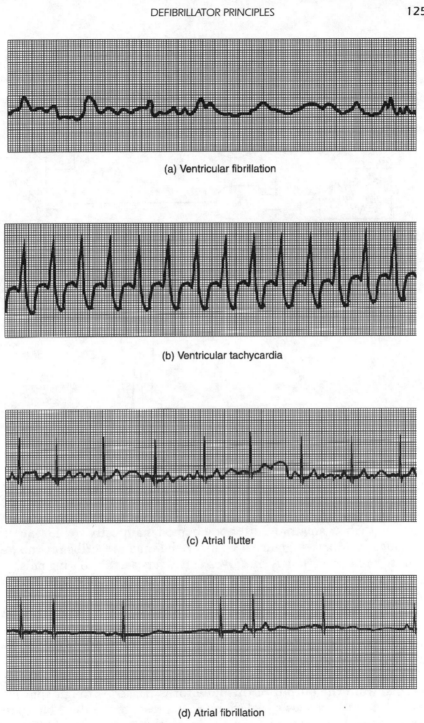

(a) Ventricular fibrillation

(b) Ventricular tachycardia

(c) Atrial flutter

(d) Atrial fibrillation

FIGURE 6.4   ECG waveforms that illustrate abnormalities (Courtesy of Nihon Koden (America) Inc.)

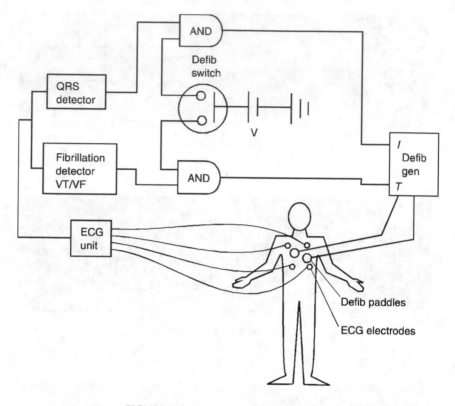

FIGURE 6.5   A diagnostic defibrillator

Cardioverter

When a physician diagnoses evidence of an abnormal supra-ventricular rhythm, such as an atrial flutter or a hemodynamically stable ventricular tachycardia (see Figure 6.4), he or she may prescribe for the patient to be cardioverted. A *cardioverter* delivers a defibrillating pulse to the heart synchronized on the R wave so that it does not accidentally cause ventricular fibrillation.

The cardioverter is attached to the patient as shown in the block diagram in Figure 6.7. Here, the leads are placed in the standard position on the chest, and the defibrillator paddles or adhesive electrodes are placed appropriately. The ECG from the patient is amplified by the ECG unit and presented to the QRS detector. When the QRS is present, a signal from the output of the detector is passed through approximately 30 milliseconds of delay and then presented to the AND gate. If the attendant is holding down the cardiovert switch, the AND gate will trigger the defibrillator pulse generator. It then defibrillates the heart approximately 30 milliseconds after the QRS. This is the point in

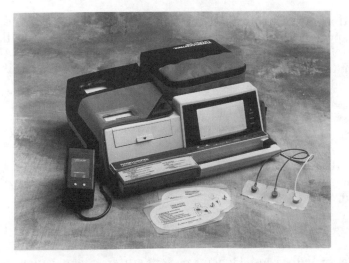

FIGURE 6.6 An automatic advisory defibrillator. Disposable defibrillator electrodes appear on the right. (Courtesy of Physiocontrol)

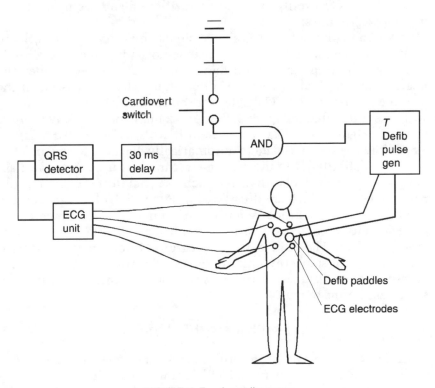

FIGURE 6.7 A cardioverter

time that the heart normally depolarizes; and delivering the defibrillating pulse at that time, should not cause the heart to fibrillate. The timing is important to keep the current pulse from hitting the heart during the *T* wave, when the ventricle may become partially depolarized and cause the heart to fibrillate.

USING AN EXTERNAL DEFIBRILLATOR

Defibrillators are designed either to be used externally or to be implanted. In this section, the use of the external defibrillator will be discussed.

Indications for Using an External Defibrillator

The defibrillator is used when a patient suffers a ventricular fibrillation (VF) or a ventricular tachycardia (VT), which leaves the patient pulseless. To verify the arrest status of the patient, institute the basic cardiopulmonary resuscitation (CPR) steps and determine the absence of breathing and circulation. When a defibrillator becomes available, check the ECG to verify ventricular fibrillation and begin ACLS (advanced cardiac life support).

When applying the ECG leads, check the leads for wet gel and make sure there is good contact because noise due to high electrode resistance could appear as a fibrillation on the display, even when the heart is normal. Make sure the expiration date has not passed on the electrodes. Check the ECG display for the characteristic VF waveform, which is illustrated in Figure 6.4(a). An example of a VT waveform is shown in Figure 6.4(b). Diagnostic defibrillators, as illustrated in Figure 6.5, would use the ECG data to automatically diagnose for VT or VF.

The defibrillator in the cardioverter mode is used to convert abnormal supra-ventricular rhythms such as atrial flutter and atrial fibrillation both of which are illustrated in Figure 6.4, observable on the ECG display. Asynchronous defibrillation may also be indicated for patients with hemodynamically unstable (systolic blood pressure of less than 90 mmHg) ventricular tachycardia. Other symptoms seen in patients with unstable rhythms are those indicative of reduced cardiac output, such as dizziness, fatigue, confusion, shortness of breath, and a decreased urine output.

Using a Defibrillator

When faced with a patient in cardiac arrest, institute basic CPR measures. If a monitored patient suddenly shows VT or VF, first try a precordial thump if a defibrillator is not immediately available. The *precordial thump* is effective in evoking ventricular depolarization and is performed by delivering a sharp blow to the patient's midsternum with the side of a fist. Continue with CPR until it is determined that the patient needs electrical defibrillation. According to the American Heart Association, the ratio of the number of chest compressions to rescue breaths during one-person CPR should be 15:2. Make chest compressions at a rate of 80 to 100 per minute and keep a ventilatory rate of 12 per minute. The ratio of chest compressions to ventilations during two-person CPR should be 5:1.

Before defibrillating, it is necessary to prepare the paddles. If gel is used, a thin layer should be spread evenly over the metal surface of both paddles. If too much gel is used, it could run across the chest and provide a path for the current to short out the pulse. In this case, the shock could not get to the heart where it is needed. Also, if the gel runs up the handle of the paddles, it could cause the user to get the defibrillation shock, a potentially fatal hazard. Gel may also be applied with a gel pad for better gel control. Another alternative is the use of pre-gelled adhesive electrodes, which are individually sealed for one-time use. Make sure the gelled pads are not out-of-date or dehydrated. Dry defibrillator pads would raise the paddle–skin resistance and result in the problems discussed previously. On a male, the paddles are placed to the right of the upper sternum, just below the clavicle. This is the paddle labeled "Sternum" in Figure 6.1. The other paddle, which is labeled "Apex" in the figure, is placed to the left of the left nipple and centered over the midclavicular line. On a female, the apex paddle should not be applied to the breast. Rather, apply it to the midaxillary line (in line with the armpit) or the anterior axillary line. For children, smaller paddles are available. If this placement does not work, the paddles may placed with one on the chest over the heart and the other on the back opposing it. This anterior–posterior position may be necessary if the patient has an implanted defibrillator and electrodes sutured to the heart deflect the current from it.

To operate the electronic equipment, follow these steps:

1. Be certain the ECG monitor is properly connected with well-gelled electrodes.

2. Select "Defibrillation" on the defibrillation–cardioversion selector.

3. Set the energy selector to 200 J, unless instructed otherwise.

4. Activate the charge button to put the proper available energy into the storage capacitor.

5. Place the paddles on the chest in the positions just described. Make sure they are separated by at least 2 inches to prevent arc-

ing. Apply a pressure of about 30 pounds to further reduce the paddle–skin resistance. Be sure the paddles are flat against the skin.

6. Be sure that no one is touching the patient. For example, if your arms were in contact with the patient's gel-covered chest, the defibrillation current would go through your heart and could cause it to fibrillate.

7. After making a final check of the ECG monitor to verify a VF or VT signal, yell "stand clear" and push both buttons on the defibrillator paddles to deliver the shock to the patient.

8. Check the ECG monitor to determine whether the QRS complex has returned and the VF or VT have disappeared.

9. If the first attempt is unsuccessful, check the electrodes. Increase the energy setting to 300 J and repeat the treatment. A third attempt should not exceed an energy setting of 360 J, unless you are otherwise instructed by a qualified health-care provider.

10. After completing the defibrillator use, continue with CPR and emergency medications for the restoration of the pulse and breathing of the patient.

Speed in doing the procedure is essential. Defibrillation success becomes significantly less after just one minute. (For further instruction see Greco p. 60.)

The procedure for urgent cardioversion is the same as the procedure for defibrillation except for these important differences:

1. Sedate the patient with IV diazepam or midazolam if he or she is still conscious.

2. Activate the synchronizer circuit.

3. Repeat steps 4 to 7 in the defibrillation procedure.

4. Depress the discharge buttons until the shock is delivered. The electrical shock may not occur instantly since it is synchronizing with the R wave.

5. For the initial shock, deliver 50 J of energy, increasing the energy level to 100 J, 200 J, and up to 360 J.

6. If ventricular fibrillation develops, immediately turn off the synchronizer and defibrillate the patient immediately.

Complications

Misdiagnosis of the need for defibrillation risks inducing ventricular fibrillation in a patient. The T wave of the ECG cycle is most vulnerable. A shock at that point could induce VF. Misdiagnosis may be caused by a faulty ECG lead connection, which causes the presentation of a false VF signal. With less experienced health-care providers, skill in finding a pulse and poor medical judgement could be a problem as well.

The defibrillation currents can cause skin burns, which sometimes are accepted as a minor adverse effect. To prevent major skin burns, never use alcohol pads as an electrical conductor. Contraction of the skeletal muscles could also cause injury. Investigations have failed to reveal thermal damage to the heart after externally applied defibrillation. Microscopic changes in the tissue have been observed, but there have been no significant effects.

Preventive Maintenance

The defibrillator is an emergency-care instrument that must be fail-safe. The equipment is characteristically in a rough environment since it must be moved to where the patient is, whether in a vehicle, in the home, or in the hospital room. Regardless of how rugged the equipment, the reliability of the device can only be ensured by frequent testing. In some hospitals, this is done on a daily basis. Some units have built in testers. An example of the test procedure is as follows:

1. Place the paddles or electrodes in the test holder.
2. Turn on the line power.
3. Set the energy selector to a maximum.

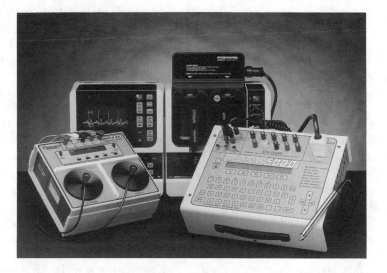

FIGURE 6.8   A defibrillator is plugged into the safety analyzer receptacle on the right. A defibrillator tester is shown on the left. (Courtesy of Dynatech Nevada, Inc.)

4. Depress the charge button.

5. Discharge the paddles or electrodes into the holder.

6. Observe the test indicator light or meter, which indicates that the proper energy has been delivered.

7. When applicable, test the battery.

The test equipment illustrated in Figure 6.8 facilitates defibrilator testing.

IMPLANTED DEFIBRILLATORS

The automatic implantable cardiac defibrillator (AICD) was first conceived of and developed by a team led by Michael Mirowski, M.D., in the 1970s. This led to clinical trials in 1980 and to approval by the Food and Drug Administration (FDA) in 1985.

Defibrillation delivered directly to the surface of the heart requires energy levels between 20 and 40 joules. This lower energy requirement allows the design of implantable defibrillators to be smaller than external devices, which need to deliver up to 400 joules externally. Current designs with batteries are contained in 10-by-10-by-2-cm packages weighing approximately 250 grams. It is approximately ten times as large as a pacemaker. The discharge capacity of the battery is sufficient for approximately 400 shocks. The monitoring lifetime of the AICD is approximately three years.

The defibrillator electrodes are sutured to the heart, as shown in Figure 6.9(a). The electrode pad is approximately 4 by 6 cm. As an alternative to the right heart patch electrode, a catheter-mounted electrode may be inserted through the superior vena cava into the mid-right atrium, as illustrated in part (b) of Figure 6.9 (see Moser). However, because of lower defibrillation thresholds, the use of two epicardial patch electrodes flanking the ventricles is an alternative. Two button-shaped sensing electrodes deliver ECG information to the defibrillator in accordance with the diagnostic schematic shown in Figure 6.5. The device constantly monitors this ECG to determine whether VT or VF is present. The VT/VF block in the figure consists of a high-pass filter that puts out a signal when a heart rate faster than the patient's highest normal sinus rhythm is present. It also measures the probability density function (PDF), the percentage of time the ECG spends at the isoelectric (zero voltage) line. When a VT or VF is present, this percentage becomes much lower than normal. If the ECG signal passes both tests, the defibrillator will be triggered to deliver a shock pulse of approximately 30 J to the heart (see Thomas).

An example of how successive shocks may be delivered is as follows: The first shock is delivered 40 seconds after the VT/VF is detected.

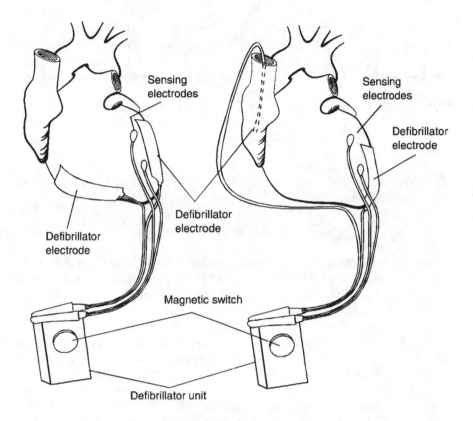

FIGURE 6.9   An AICD

Of this 40 seconds, 20 seconds is used to sense the rhythm abnormality and 5 to 15 seconds is used to charge the pulse generator. If the first attempt is unsuccessful, a second shock approximately 20 percent more intense is delivered. If it is still unsuccessful, up to four shocks are delivered, after which the AICD turns off, unless it senses a 35-second period of a "normal" rhythm that satisfies both the rate and PDF criteria. If the rhythm is still abnormal, further resuscitation would have to be done by CPR, medications, and external defibrillation.

A sample ECG recording of an arrhythmia and its conversion to normal sinus rhythm after two defibrillation shocks is shown in Figure 6.10. In this case, the normal ECG degenerates into VF. After 40 seconds, the first shock fails to convert the VF. However, 40 seconds later, it succeeds. The defibrillation pulse is normally about 700 volts and 6 ms in duration to generate the appropriate shock energy. The high energy of the shock leaks into the ECG circuit and may overload it for a time considerably longer than the 6-ms defibrillator pulse duration. The

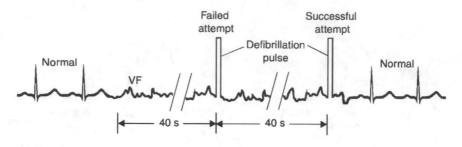

FIGURE 6.10   An ECG recording of AICD operation. (From Thomas)

ECG display would then be temporarily distorted, due to the effects of the overloaded circuits.

Implantation

The surgical electrode implantation techniques include the subxiphoid or subcostal, median sternotomy, and lateral thoracotomy approaches. AICDs are implanted via the median sternotomy approach 20 percent of the time when concomitant surgery is involved. Such surgery includes coronary artery bypass grafting, VT mapping, ventricular aneurysmectomy, or endocardial resection. If the surgeon suspects a future need for an AICD, he or she will place the patches during the concomitant procedure and place the generator at a later date.

Some prefer the lateral thoracotomy for patients with previous sternotomies. This approach minimizes the hazards of a redo sternotomy in those patients who have undergone previous cardiac procedures. Postoperative adhesions from prior surgery can be avoided, therefore lessening the danger of cardiac bypass graft or great vessel injury. This approach also allows good visualization of the heart. Unfortunately, it is associated with a large amount of pain and, therefore, a slower postoperative recovery.

As with the lateral thoracotomy, the subxiphoid or subcostal approach is undertaken in patients with previous sternotomies. Unlike the lateral thoracotomy, this approach is associated with a much easier postoperative recovery period due to a smaller incision and prompt extubation. However, because access to the heart is limited, this approach is reserved for those patients with larger-sized hearts.

Because of the size and weight of the AICD unit, it is implanted in an abdominal pocket rather than in the subclavian area that is used for pacemakers. The subcutaneous pocket is developed in the left paraumbilical area just anterior to the abdominal fascia. It makes a noticeable bulge there. The leads from the electrodes on the heart and the sensing leads are tunneled subcutaneously to the pocket and connected to the AICD terminals.

During implantation, the physician determines the defibrillating threshold using an external cardioverter/defibrillator to convert induced fibrillations. The threshold may be as high as 40 J. The frequency of the patient's tachycardia is used to determine the cutoff frequency of the VT and VF detector. Cutoff frequencies from 120 to 200 bpm are available. The physician chooses a cutoff rate below the patient's known tachycardia, but above the highest normal sinus rhythm. This ensures that the patient will not receive a shock during strenuous labor, when under emotional stress, or during times of excitement.

Indications for Implantation

The FDA has approved two classes of patients for AICD: (1) those who have survived at least one cardiac arrest not associated with acute myocardial infarction (MI) and (2) those who, in the absence of a previous arrest, have experienced VF or VT or both and who can be induced into VT or VF, which causes pulselessness that cannot be controlled with drug therapy. Most patients who receive an AICD can be induced into VT or VF in spite of the use of antiarrhythmic medications. However, since the AICD does not prevent arrhythmias, antiarrhythmic medications will also be prescribed to reduce the incidence of arrhythmias.

There are several cases where a patient would not be a candidate for an AICD. Patients with ventricular arrhythmias from transient causes, such as a recent MI, drug toxicity, drowning, electrocution, electrolyte imbalances, and hypoxia, are not candidates for an AICD. Patients who have frequent episodes of VT or VF are not candidates because the frequent shocks may be painful and cause intolerable anxiety for the patient. Furthermore, frequent surgery for battery changes due to excessive use of the device may impose further risk of surgical complications and financial stress. Patients who express extreme psychological resistance to the device or who are not expected to survive another 12 months may be denied an AICD implantation. Patients with unipolar pacemakers may not receive an AICD because the pacing pulse interferes with the defibrillator. Bipolar pacemakers are usually compatible with an AICD.

AICD patients have been shown to have survival rates of 98.2 percent after one year (Thomas). This is up from survival rates as low as 50 percent in the first year for people for whom antiarrhythmic agents are not effective.

Complications

Complications with the AICD can be placed into two major categories: (1) complications associated with the surgery or (2) complications with the function of the device.

Surgical mortality is estimated at 2 percent and is primarily due to underlying cardiopulmonary disease and the concomitant surgery performed with AICD implantation. As with any cardiac surgery, the potential postoperative problems include the development of bleeding, pericardial effusions, pericarditis, pneumothorax, and pneumonia, as well as other respiratory complications. Although prophylactic intravenous antibiotics are administered, infection still occurs in about 4 percent of the cases and may range from a generator site cellulitis to a severe mediastinitis. An infection may require the removal of the leads, electrodes, and defibrillator; however, aggressive antibiotic therapy has decreased the incidence of device explantation to 2 percent.

Postoperative arrhythmias, such as sinus tachycardia and atrial arrhythmia, may cause false-positive shocks. These may be frequent enough that the AICD must be temporarily turned off and other treatments used to deal with this transient phenomenon. This saves the battery, which is capable of approximately 400 shocks. Also, the shocks cause pain and discomfort to the patient and heighten his or her anxiety about the device.

In 2 percent of the patients, device malfunction results from a fracture in the bipolar rate-sensing lead. This may result in inappropriate shocks and require surgical intervention.

Electromagnetic radiation from devices like airport security systems, magnetic resonance imagers (MRIs), electrical surgical units (ESUs), and pacemakers could interfere with the AICD.

Postoperative Nursing Implications

The postoperative care of AICD patients is similar to the care received by other patients requiring cardio-thoracic surgery. Vital signs (heart rate and rhythm, blood pressure, and temperature), chest tube drainage, and respiratory status (arterial blood gasses and breath sounds) are monitored frequently. The incisions are assessed for bleeding as well as for signs of infection. Extubation coughing, deep breathing, and early mobilization are encouraged to decrease the incidence of common pulmonary complications, such as atelectasis and pneumonia. The use of pain medications should be encouraged prior to activities or procedures. Adequate pain control will allow the patient to mobilize early and prevent pulmonary complications.

In addition to the postoperative care given to cardio-thoracic surgical patients, there are special considerations specific to the AICD patient. Since these patients are already prone to malignant arrhythmias, common postoperative factors that increase cardiac irritability may further predispose them to a lethal event. Therefore, the nurse must continually assess the patient for and correct electrolyte and acid/base imbalances, hemodynamic instability, hypoxia, and hypercapnia. The nurse must also be cognizant of other factors that promote the development of electrical instability, such as manipulation of the heart during surgery, discontinuation of antiarrhythmic medications, pericarditis, and intracardiac catheters.

Because arrhythmias are common in these patients, the nurse should confirm the active or inactive status of the AICD and the manner in which it functions. The AICD is activated or deactivated with a magnet. To activate some AICDs, you place the magnet directly over the unit and listen for a beeping tone. When the beeping tone becomes synchronized with the *QRS* complex, the AICD is activated. To deactivate it, you place the magnet over the AICD generator and listen for a continuous tone.

Some institutions keep the AICD inactive for the first 24 to 72 hours after implantation. This will avoid the inappropriate shocks from the AICD in response to the common supraventricular arrhythmias encountered in the immediate postoperative period. If the patient experiences VT or VF while the AICD is inactive, it will not be able to sense or respond to the arrhythmia. Emergency procedures such as external defibrillation should be undertaken immediately. The AICD will remain undamaged by external defibrillation unless the defibrillator paddles are placed directly over the generator. If the anterior–lateral position of the paddles is unsuccessful, attempt the anterior–posterior paddle placement.

When the AICD is in the active mode, it should defibrillate the patient. If the patient is conscious during a life-threatening arrhythmia, monitor the patient and the ECG, and allow the AICD to defibrillate. If the device fails to defibrillate or if the arrhythmia is not terminated by the AICD, institute emergency measures immediately and defibrillate externally. Be aware that while the AICD is discharging, a slight harmless but startling tingle may be felt by someone touching the patient. To insulate yourself from this feeling, wear rubber gloves while performing CPR.

Psychosocial Concerns

Feelings of fear and anxiety are common problems associated with AICD patients. During the hospitalization, patients are anxious regarding the diagnostic process and treatment regime. These patients undergo electrophysiologic (EP) testing to ensure that the AICD will function appropriately. During the EP studies, the lethal arrhythmia is induced and the AICD is allowed to fire and terminate the arrhythmia. These studies, which at times need to be repeated, are dreaded by patients. Many are fearful of the pain the AICD will cause as it defibrillates, while others fear the AICD will not be able to terminate the arrhythmia. During the hospitalization, the nurse should provide time for the patient and family to verbalize their feelings and express their questions and concerns. To allay fears of pain during AICD defibrillation, explain that some patients say that it feels like a punch or kick to the chest, while others describe only a slight discomfort. The EP studies may also reduce the patient's fears regarding AICD discharge because they will be able to experience a defibrillation in a controlled setting.

Many patients are anxious about leaving the hospital where 24-hour nursing exists. Many feel helpless since their lives depend on a machine. They express a concern that the AICD will interfere with their quality of life. They fear AICD firing and misfiring and, because of this, are reluctant to be left alone or may even be afraid to go out in public because they don't want to "make a scene." Fortunately, the nurse can reassure the patient that a productive life can be resumed after AICD implantation. Most patients employed before the AICD implantation resume work after the surgery. Other physical restrictions are similar to those of typical cardiac surgery patients. In addition, activities that involve direct contact with the generator should be avoided. Also, patients will be advised not to drive for about six months postoperatively to avoid a potential accident that may occur because of an arrhythmia. Some patients will not ever be able to drive an automobile or work in precarious places, such as on ladders and scaffolds, if they have been known to lose consciousness even with the firing of the AICD.

To aid in the patient's and family's adaptation to the AICD, many institutions have developed support groups. The support groups will enable patients and their families to share their experiences. This will assist the newer AICD patients in overcoming their fears and provide continued support for all involved in the group.

Educational Needs

Patients and their families will have many learning needs because of the complexity of the AICD. They will need specific information about the AICD device and how it functions, their postoperative rehabilitation and life-style, activity level and restrictions, medications, and follow-up care. An example regiment is illustrated in the chart shown in Box 6.1. It is also recommended that the family be trained in CPR.

Postoperative teaching should begin once the patient is stable. Instructions should be simple, clear, detailed, and specific. Both verbal and written information should be presented. To enhance learning, booklets and videotapes are available from the manufacturer. To ensure effective learning, simplicity, repetition, and review are needed. Adequate time should be allowed to pursue and encourage questions. Many patients have misconceptions about their AICD, thinking that it will cure their underlying heart disease. These erroneous assumptions should be clarified as soon as possible. Because the patient requires lifelong follow-up care, he or she must have an adequate understanding of the information.

BOX 6.1

Follow-up Care/Patient Teaching Chart

General Information

The AICD is an implantable device capable of delivering up to five shocks if it senses a dangerous, abnormal rhythm (ventricular tachycardia or ventricular fibrillation).

Bathing

The patient may begin showers about one week postoperatively and tub baths three weeks after surgery.

Cardiopulmonary Resuscitation

Immediate family members must know CPR.

Clothing

To prevent chafing the skin over the AICD generator, tight or restrictive clothing should be avoided.

Driving

Your specific medical condition and physician will determine whether driving is permitted. Driving restrictions exist in some states regarding patients that may lose consciousness.

Electrical Considerations

Most household appliances will not interfere with the AICD. Any surgical procedure involving electrosurgery requires the deactivation of the AICD.

Electromagnetic Considerations

Strong magnetic fields, such as large transformers, radio-frequency transmitters, arc welders, and MRIs, may cause inappropriate discharge or inhibit the sensing of the AICD. Stay at least two feet away from the alternators of power lawn mowers, boats, or cars. AICDs have a warning sound, such as a beeping tone, when it interacts with a magnetic field. It may be inactivated if you remain near the magnetic field for a prolonged period of time. Leave the area and contact the M.D./R.N. responsible for your follow-up care. He or she may need to reactivate the device.

(continued)

BOX 6.1

Follow-Up Care/Patient Teaching Chart (continued)

Incision/Wound Care

Incisions should be cleaned daily with soap and water. The generator site should be checked daily for signs of infection. A fever or any signs of infection should be reported.

Lifting

The patient should not lift more than ten pounds or perform isometric exercises for four to six weeks postoperatively to allow adequate incision healing. Isometric exercises include mowing the lawn and vacuuming.

Medic Alert

Wear a Medic Alert bracelet or necklace and carry a manufacturer's AICD identification card.

Recreation

The patient should avoid activities that have direct contact with the generator site. An ECG stress test should be obtained before beginning strenuous exercise. The pulse should be monitored before and after any exercise.

Sex

Sexual activity is not restricted. However, the patient should avoid positions that would place stress on the incisions.

Shocks

The patient should report all shocks. If two shocks occur within a short time, the patient should go to the hospital to have the device examined. The patient should keep a diary of when and how many shocks were received and of symptoms and activities before, during, and after the shocks. If the patient continues to feel aftershocks, the paramedics should be called and the patient should lie down. When the paramedics arrive, they should be told immediately about the AICD.

(continued)

BOX 6.1

Follow-Up Care/Patient Teaching Chart (continued)

Travel

Travel is not restricted. The AICD may trigger metal detectors at airports, but it won't be harmed by them. However, prolonged exposure to the magnetic wand, also used for security at airports, may deactivate the AICD. The patient should keep an AICD identification card to present to airport security.

Adapted from Higgins, C.

Follow-Up Care

Patients are seen one or two weeks after discharge to reinforce discharge medications and instructions and to assess incision sites. After that, the patients are seen for follow-up device checks every two months for the first year and monthly thereafter. Patients are also taught to notify their physician immediately after receiving a shock. If several shocks are received, hospitalization may be necessary to stabilize the heart rhythm. During the patient's monthly visits, a defibrillator self-testing device, AIDCHECK, evaluates the battery life of the AICD. The AIDCHECK also displays a pulse count that keeps track of the number of times the device has discharged.

REFERENCES

American Heart Association, "Guidelines for Cardiopulmonary Resuscitation and Emergency Cardiac Care." *Journal of the American Medical Association* 268, no. 16 (1992): 2171–2295.

Aston, R. *Principles of Biomedical Instrumentation and Measurement.* Riverside, NJ: Macmillan Publishing Co., 1990: Chapter 8.

Chapman, P. "The Implantable Defibrillator and the Emergency Physician." *Annals of Emergency Medicine* 18, no. 5 (1989): 579–81.

Crockett, R. J., B. M. Droppet, and S. E. Higgins. *Defibrillation: What You Should Know.* Redmond, WA: Physio-Control, 1991.

Damiano, R., et al. "Implantation of Cardioverter Defibrillators in the Post-Sternotomy Patient." *Annals of Thoracic Surgery* 53, (1992): 978–83.

DeBorde, R., D. Aarons, and M. Biggs. "The Automatic Implantable Cardioverter." *AACN's Clinical Issues in Critical Care Nursing* 2, no. 1 (1991): 170–77.

Greco, A. "An Expert's Guide to Using a Defibrillator." *Nursing* 17, no. 8 (August 1987): 60–63.

Health Care Provider's Manual for Basic Life Support. Dallas: American Heart Association, 1988.

Higgins, C. "The AICD: A Teaching Plan for Patients and Families." *Critical Care Nurse* 10, no. 6 (1990): 69–74.

Lee, B. L., and G. Mirabal. "Automatic Implantable Cardioverter Defibrillator." *Association of Operating Room Nurses (AORN) Journal* 50, no. 6 (December 1989): 1218–27.

Manolis, A., H. Rastegar, and M. Estes. "Automatic Implantable Cardioverter Defibrillator." *Journal of the American Medical Association* 262, no. 10 (1989): 1362–67.

McCrum, A., and A. Tyndall. "Nursing Care for Patients With Implantable Defibrillators." *Critical Care Nurse* 9, no. 9 (1989): 48–66.

Miller, K. M. "When Your Patient has an Implanted Defibrillator." *RN Magazine* 53, no. 6 (June 1990): 32–35.

Mirowski, M. "The Implantable Cardioverter-Defibrillator." *The Heart.* Edited by J. Hurst et al. New York: McGraw-Hill, 1990: 2110–12.

Moser, S. A., et al. "Caring for Patients with Implantable Cardioverter Defibrillators." *Critical Care Nurse* 8, no. 2 (March/April 1988): 52–62.

Opalden, J. "Automatic Implantable Cardioverter Defibrillators." *Nursing90* 20, no. 5 (May 1990): 64G–64M.

Paris, P. M. "EMT-Defibrillation: A Recipe for Saving Lives." *American Journal of Emergency Medicine* 6 (1988): 282–87.

Schuster, D. "Patients With an Implanted Cardioverter Defibrillator: A New Challenge." *Journal of Emergency Nursing* 16, no. 3 (1990): 219–25.

Textbook of Advanced Cardiac Life Support. 2nd ed. Dallas: American Heart Association, 1987.

Thomas, Andra. "Automatic Implantable Cardioverter-Defibrillator." *Journal of Cardiovascular Nursing* 3, no. 1 (November 1988): 77–87.

Weaver, W. D., et al. "Use of the Automated External Defibrillator in the Management of Out-of-hospital Cardiac Arrest." *New England Journal of Medicine* 319 (1988): 661–66.

EXERCISES

1. Define a defibrillator.
2. Within what range of currents, applied to two different limbs, will the heart be apt to fibrillate?
3. What has changed since the early defibrillators of the 1950s to improve their reliability?
4. Why is accurate diagnosis of a fibrillating heart critical?
5. After what period of time does the likelihood of reversing a fibrillation of the heart with a defibrillator rapidly decline?

6. How does the diagnostic defibrillator increase the effectiveness of the defibrillator?

7. In what circuit component of a Lown defibrillator is the energy available to defibrillate the patient stored?

8. Why is it necessary to charge the capacitor in a defibrillator?

9. A defibrillator has a 16 μF storage capacitor. If it is charged up to 3,000 V, how much energy is stored in it?

10. Name three symptoms of a fibrillating heart that can be observed without the aid of instrumentation.

11. Sketch the ECG waveform characteristic of a heart fibrillation.

12. What is the approximate frequency of oscillation of a fibrillating waveform?

13. Draw the block diagram of a diagnostic defibrillator.

14. What distinctive feature of an ECG indicates that the heart is not fibrillating?

15. What two features of an ECG would indicate that the heart is fibrillating?

16. Under what conditions is a cardioverter used?

17. Why is cardioversion not an emergency procedure?

18. Why does the defibrillation pulse used for cardioversion need to be timed to flow 30 ms after the QRS complex?

19. What could be the effect if a normally contracting ventricle is hit with a defibrillator pulse during the T wave?

20. How is the available energy stored in the capacitor distributed when it is released into a patient?

21. What range of energies is a typical external defibrillator able to deliver to the paddles and thorax?

22. A defibrillator has an available energy of 300 joules. If the thorax resistance is 50 ohms, the electrode–skin resistance of the paddle is 40 ohms, and the internal resistance of the defibrillator is 10 ohms, what is the energy (in joules) distributed throughout the thorax?

23. What is the effect on the patient if the paddle does not have sufficient gel?

24. How could high electrode–skin resistance result in a false indication of ventricular fibrillation on an ECG trace?

25. Name two conditions that indicate the use of an external defibrillator.

26. How do you check a patient for consciousness?

27. How do you check a patient for breathing?

28. How do you check a patient for a pulse?

29. What condition indicates the need for cardioversion?

30. Why is too little gel on the paddles a hazard to the patient?

31. How could too much gel on the paddle be a hazard to the operator?

32. How could too much gel be a hazard to the patient?

33. Name two positions for external defibrillator paddles.

34. Why should an ECG be used before a patient is defibrillated?

35. By what distance should the defibrillator paddles be separated?

36. How much pressure is needed on gelled metal defibrillator electrodes?

37. How does one determine that the defibrillation was successful?

38. What is the risk to the patient if VF is wrongly diagnosed?

39. What could cause a false fibrillation trace on the ECG?

40. Does external defibrillation cause damage to the heart muscle?

41. Who invented the first AICD?

42. When was the AICD first approved by the FDA?

43. What energy levels are required to defibrillate a heart when the electrodes are implanted in it?

44. What is the approximate weight of an AICD?

45. How many defibrillation pulses can a typical AICD deliver?

46. Describe two positions for the defibrillator electrodes on the AICD.

47. What is the function of the sensing electrode on the AICD?

48. Identify three surgical approaches to AICD implantation.

49. Why would the AICD be implanted in the paraumbilical area?

50. How is the cutoff rate of the VF and VT detector in the AICD determined?

51. How do you ensure that the AICD does not shock the patient during strenuous exercise?

52. What are the approved FDA classifications for AICD candidates?

53. Why would a person with frequent VT or VF not be a candidate for AICD implantation?

54. What type of pacemaker lead is compatible with an AICD unit?

55. What is the one-year survival rate for AICD patients?

56. How are frequent postoperative arrhythmias due to AICD implantation treated?

57. List four complications that are possible after AICD implantation.

Pacemakers and TENS Devices

The concept of pacing the heart with an electrical pulse of current was demonstrated by Albert S. Hymen, an American cardiologist, in 1932. However, the first clinical use of the concept was made by Paul M. Zoll when he applied a current to the surface of the skin in 1952, thus starting external cardiac pacing. The advent of the transistor in the 1950s made the fully implantable pacemaker possible, because the transistor is much smaller, uses far less energy, and runs cooler than the vacuum tube it replaced. On the suggestion of Dr. Simon Rodbard of the Chronic Disease Research Institute in Buffalo, New York, Wilson Greatbatch, an American engineer, invented the pacing circuit. Greatbatch enthusiastically promoted his idea until he got American physicians William Chardak and Andrew Gage to utilize his circuit in the first clinically successful pacemaker, implanted in 1960. This pacemaker dramatically demonstrated how effective machines could be in delivering therapy, by saving the lives of many people suffering from complete heart block (Stoke-Adams syndrome) when all other therapeutic options had failed.

This was the first artificial spare part for the heart. Others followed such as artificial heart valves, culminating in the artificial heart implanted in a dentist, Barney Clark, by William DeVries in 1982. This implant, the Jarvik-7, designed by Robert K. Jarvik, was initially intended for permanent implantation, but it is now considered an emergency bridge until heart transplantation can be achieved. Serious problems with the artificial heart discouraging its permanent use are the lack of an implantable power source, and clotting and hemolysis of the blood caused by the mechanical structure.

The early pacemaker was a simple prosthesis intended to replace the function of either a diseased sinoatrial (SA) node of the heart or the atrioventricular (AV) node. It was capable of curing the bradycardia that results when the normal pacing pulse from the SA node does not reach the ventricle and the muscle beats at its own slow rate of around 40 bpm.

PACEMAKER BASICS

The simplest pacemaker consists of four elements, which are illustrated in the block diagram in Figure 7.1. These are a digital pulse generator, a catheter to the heart ventricle, an electrode in contact with the ventricle, and a battery.

The *digital pulse generator* produces a stimulus of voltage that has a level ranging up to approximately 5 V. The pulse has a duration, T_D, ranging from 0.1 to 2.3 ms for each beat of the heart, as illustrated in Figure 7.2. This pulse travels along an insulated wire passing through a *catheter* into the patient's heart atrium or ventricle. The wire delivers a current produced by the voltage pulse to an *electrode* attached to the cardiac muscle. This electrode serves as an alternative stimulus site for the heartbeat. The electrical resistance of the electrode–muscle interface, R_H, may range from 100 to 1,400 ohms, depending on the type of contact and tissue morphology. When R_H is high, one would need more voltage to drive an adequate stimulus current into the heart tissue. The return path of the current is through the body viscera to one terminal of the battery, which is attached to the metal casing of the pacemaker. The other terminal of the battery then provides voltage to the digital pulse oscillator to complete the stimulus circuit.

A typical stimulus pulse level is shown in Figure 7.3. This is a stimulus-duration curve. The longer the stimulus, the lower the stimulus level may be. Because the battery stores a fixed amount of energy, the energy of the stimulus is crucial in determining the battery lifetime

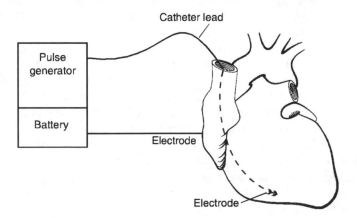

FIGURE 7.1   A pacemaker block diagram

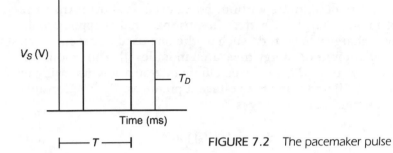

FIGURE 7.2   The pacemaker pulse

of the pacemaker. When it is used up, the pacemaker battery must be replaced by surgery.

The Pacemaker Battery

Finding a battery that was small enough and that stored enough energy to run a pacemaker for years at a time without changing was a major task for the early developers of implantable pacemakers. At first, mercury cell batteries, which could last for about two years, were used. Further development has lead to lithium-iodide batteries, which can last as long as fifteen years without being replaced.

This long lifetime is due to the fact that pacemakers are made with complementary-metal-oxide semiconductors (CMOS). This means that the metal input conductor is separated from the semiconductor circuit by an extremely thin silicon dioxide film. Silicon dioxide is glass and a very good insulator. Therefore, the CMOS chips take very little current from the battery that supplies them with energy; as a result, the batteries last for a long time. In fact, they last so long that it usually does not help to use rechargeable batteries in a pacemaker. Rechargeable batteries can be recharged from outside the body. However, the shelf life of a rechargeable battery, or the time that it takes

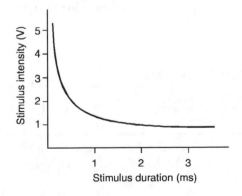

FIGURE 7.3   The stimulation threshold plotted against the pulse width. (From Citron, P., et. al. "Cardiac Pacing," in Therapeutic Medical Devices: Application and Design, Cook and Webster, eds., © 1982, p. 46. Reprinted by permission of Prentice Hall, Englewood Cliffs, NJ)

for the battery to deteriorate without being used, is shorter than the lifetime of a nonrechargeable battery in most pacemaker applications.

A nonrechargeable battery, such as the one used in pacemakers, stores a fixed amount of energy measured in joules (J). The amount of energy a battery stores, E_B, can be calculated if you know its rating in ampere-hour (A-H) units, and the voltage it produces, V_B. The formula for calculating this stored energy is

$$E_B = 3,600 \, (A\text{-}H)(V_B) \text{ joules} \tag{7.1}$$

Here, the units on A-H are ampere-hours and on V_B are volts. A dimensional analysis of this formula to the right of the equals sign is

$$\left(\frac{3,600 \text{ sec}}{\text{hour}} \right) (\text{ampere-hour}) (\text{volt})$$
$$= (\text{watt-second})$$
$$= \left(\frac{\text{joules}}{\text{second}} \right) (\text{second})$$
$$= \text{joules}$$

Here 3,600 seconds are recognized to be in one hour. Also, the power used by an element equals the volts across it times the amperes through it and is measured in watts. Furthermore, the watts of power have units of joules per second. Then the second units cancel and you end up with units of joules.

Typically, the batteries used in a pacemaker have a capacity ranging from 0.44 to 3.2 A-H. The limitation on battery capacity is the size, which increases in proportion to the capacity. Also, the shelf life of the battery limits its lifetime. Thus, a capacity that would last longer than the battery shelf life would be wasted, because the battery would deteriorate before it could be used.

EXAMPLE 7.1   A pacemaker battery is rated at 2 A-H. The battery terminal voltage is 1.5 V. How much energy is available from this battery?

Solution   Using Equation (7.1), you have

$$E_B = 3,600(2)1.5 = 10,800 \text{ J}$$

Example 7.2 shows what the lifetime of this battery might be.

EXAMPLE 7.2   Suppose a pacing pulse required to capture the heartbeat contains 10 microjoules of energy. If the heart is paced at 70 bpm, how long will the battery described in Example 7.1 last?

Solution From the previous example, you see that the battery stores 10,800 J of energy. At 10 µJ per beat, you have

$$\text{Number of beats} = \frac{10,800}{10\,(10)^{-6}} \text{ beats}$$

At the rate of 70 bpm, the lifetime in minutes is

$$\text{Lifetime} = 1,080 \times 10^6 \frac{\text{beat}}{70 \text{ beat/min}} = 15.43 \times 10^6 \text{ min}$$

Converting this to years gives

$$\text{Lifetime} = (15.43 \times 10^6 \text{ min}) \frac{1\,\text{h}}{60\,\text{min}} \frac{1\,\text{yr}}{8760\,\text{h}} = 29.35 \text{ yr}$$

This example shows a maximum lifetime. The actual battery lifetime would be shortened if the pacing energy requirement for each pulse were higher, if the electrode resistance were increased, if more than one chamber of the heart were paced, and if the pulse rate were higher. Also, the battery will deteriorate from aging factors, again shortening the lifetime. A battery is made of toxic materials. Therefore, every precaution must be used in its design to prevent it from rupturing and releasing these materials into the body. The care giver should prepare to answer patient questions such as "How old is my battery?" with an answer like: This information is available from the manufacturing date of the pacemaker, since the battery is integral to the pacemaker package. If the patient asks "How do I know my battery is getting weak?" review the testing procedures, and indicate the importance of looking for end-of-life signs listed by the manufacturer. If the patient wonders if the battery would corrode, give assurance that the pacemaker is designed and tested to be biocompatable.

Pacemaker Properties

Pacemakers are characterized by a set of parameters defined as follows:

Rate—The range of beats per minute, typically adjustable from 25 to 150 bpm.

Sensitivity—The extent to which a pacemaker is responsive to levels of electrical activity in the heart. That is, the voltage feedback from the patient's heart, conducted through a lead, needed to control the pacemaker's performance. Typical values range from 0.7 to 5.5 mV.

Pulse width—The time duration of the stimulus pulse, shown as T_D in Figure 7.2. The typical range is from 0.1 to 2.3 ms.

Pulse amplitude—The stimulus voltage level delivered by the pacemaker, as illustrated in Figure 7.2. The typical range is from 2.5 to 10 V.

Battery capacity—A measure of the storage capacity of a battery, rated in ampere-hours (A-H). One A-H means the battery would be able to deliver one ampere of current for one hour before it becomes depleted. Typical pacemakers require an A-H from 0.44 to 3.2 A-H.

Longevity—The lifetime of the pacemaker before a battery change is required. The typical lifetime is from 3.5 to 18 years.

End-of-life indicator—The signal given by the pacemaker that the battery is getting weak. This may be a 2- to 10-percent drop in pulse rate or a diagnostic signal measurable during testing.

Size—The volume of the pacemaker, typically ranging from 22 to 80 cm^3.

Weight—The weight of the pacing unit, excluding the leads. The typical range is from 33 to 98 gm (1.2 to 3.5 oz).

Encapsulation material—The biologically compatible material that encloses the pacemaker circuit and battery and prevents leakage into the body fluids. The materials used are silicon rubber, titanium, and stainless steel.

Unipolar lead—A pacemaker lead having a single electrode attached to the heart. The pacing current exits that electrode into the heart and returns to the battery through the conductive body fluids and viscera. This has the advantage of having only one wire and one electrode, therefore it is simpler and uses less hardware.

Bipolar lead—A pacemaker lead consisting of two wires through one catheter, each attached to a separate electrode. The stimulus current exits one electrode and returns through the second electrode a few centimeters behind it. This has the advantage of confining the stimulus current to the region between the two electrodes. This tends to reduce susceptibility to interference from stray electric and magnetic fields which could cause arrhythmias.

In an *endocardial* configuration, the pacemaker leads are usually passed through a catheter into the right atrium or right ventricle of the heart, as illustrated in Figure 7.4(a). The catheter is passed into a major vein in one of these chambers in a relatively simple surgical procedure. The pacing electrode is connected to a beating heart, which tends to create a relative motion between the tissue and electrode. If

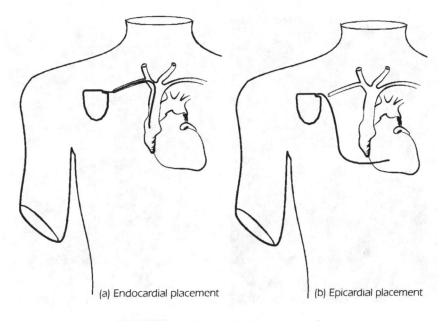

(a) Endocardial placement   (b) Epicardial placement

FIGURE 7.4   Pacemaker lead connections

the lead is lodged in the RV, it is fitted with tines that lock themselves into the Purkinje muscle fibers, as illustrated in Figure 7.5(a). This keeps it in place as the heart beats. It also helps if the lead has a porous tip, as illustrated in Figure 7.5(b). This reduces the relative motion between the tip and the wall of the heart, keeping the electrode resistance (due to scar buildup) low. Another method of attaching the lead is by screwing a helical wire into the heart muscle. If, on the other hand, the lead is lodged in the atrium, the lead tip is bent into the shape of the letter "J", appropriately called a *J-electrode* and shown in Figure 7.5(c). This connects to the atrial muscle, conforming to the chamber walls.

Although the endocardial lead is most commonly used, an *epicardial lead* may also be used. In this case, the lead is sutured to the external wall of the heart, as illustrated in Figure 7.4(b), during open-heart surgery. During open-heart surgery, while the myocardial surface is visible, the epicardial leads (atrial and ventricular) can easily be placed to facilitate temporary pacing. During the immediate postoperative period they can also be utilized in the diagnosis and treatment of postoperative dysrhythmia. The atrial leads can be hooked up to an ECG machine to perform an atrial electrocardiogram. This type of ECG looks at atrial electrical activity and how it relates to ventricular electrical activity. The atrial electrocardiogram helps to identify various dysrhythmia that are difficult to interpret with standard electrocardiograms. Pacemakers that suppress tachycardia and ventricular fibrillations may require an epicardial lead or patch.

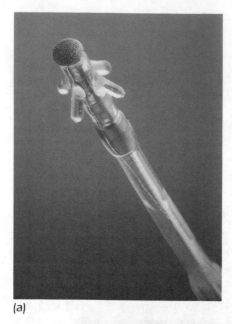

(a)

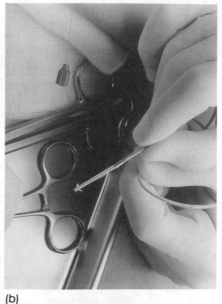

(b)

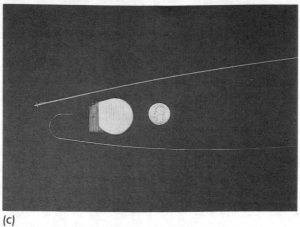

(c)

FIGURE 7.5 Endocardial pacemaker leads. (a) A steroid-eluting cardiac pacing lead (Courtesy of Medtronic Inc.). (b) A tined bipolar lead
(Courtesy of Medtronic Inc.). (c) The J- and tined electrodes shown next
to a pacemaker, with a quarter as a size reference.

Changes in the electrode–tissue contact naturally occur over
time. The pacemaker electrode rubs the endocardial surface and causes
those cells in contact with the electrode to become injured. This
trauma results in acute inflammation and subsequent fibrin deposition.
Physiologically, this results in the formation of fibrous scar tissue (up

to 2 mm in thickness). Electrically, this results in increased resistance and polarization voltage buildup. Therefore, a stimulus voltage chosen at implantation may not be adequate to supply sufficient stimulus current to pace the heart after a time. Even the simplest programmable pacemakers allow an external adjustment of the stimulus level to correct for this aging effect.

Tissue scarring and electrode separation are minimized by the tined and J-electrode leads. The polarization due to ionic current flow can be reduced by use of a *biphasic* pulse. In this case, every successive pulse drives the current in an opposite direction. Thus, the polarization left from one pulse will be cancelled by the following pulse.

Programmable Pacemakers

Because of the aging effects in the pacemaker–patient interface, it is desirable that pacemakers have a programming capability, at least for stimulus adjustment. For example, if, to compensate for aging, one increased the stimulus level at implantation time, a shorter battery lifetime would result. The simplest pacemaker is the asynchronous device illustrated in Figure 7.6(a). Here, a single lead is passed through a catheter into the ventricle of the heart. *Asynchronous* means that the pacemaker is not synchronized and beats at its own preset rate regardless of the heart activity. Programming to change the stimulus parameters can be achieved on the implanted pacemaker by the use of a magnetic switch. The switch position is changed by placing a magnet on the skin of the patient just above the implanted pacemaker. Digital codes are then used to select the stimulus level, pulse duration, and rate in beats per minute.

In addition to programming the stimulus parameters, it is possible to change the circuit configuration from outside the body, or during implantation, on some programmable pacemakers. For example, the magnetic switch can be used to convert the pacemaker from an asynchronous type to an *R* wave inhibited type. An *R wave inhibited* pacemaker will be turned off by the presence of an *R* wave from the heart's depolarization. Because the pacing lead can sense the *R* wave, a different set of leads to the heart is not required. Therefore, the change can be made while the pacemaker is implanted.

On this pacemaker, if the *R* wave does not appear after a preset period, the pacer will deliver a stimulus. This is called a *demand pacemaker*, because the stimulus is not delivered unless there is a demand for it. This has the advantage of allowing the heart to function normally when it will and saving battery energy as well.

A third alternative circuit, illustrated in part (c) of Figure 7.6, is a *P* wave synchronous, as selected by the magnetic switch. The *P wave synchronous* configuration delivers a stimulus to the ventricle a fixed

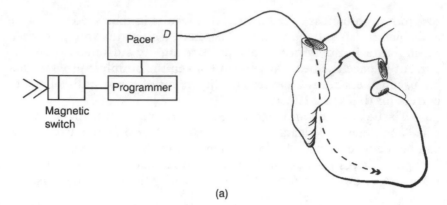

(a)

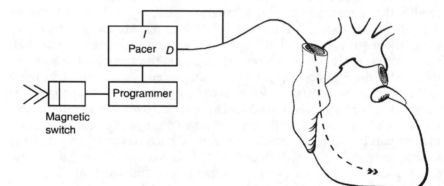

(b)

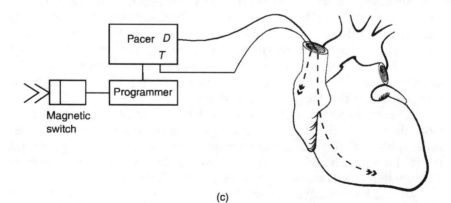

(c)

FIGURE 7.6   Programmable pacemakers

time after it has sensed the *P* wave through a lead attached to the atrium. The sensitivity parameter specified for the pacemaker identifies the minimum value of feedback from the atrium necessary to trigger it. Two leads are necessary, so if they were not present at implantation, this mode could not be chosen later. However, when the two leads are in place, one could choose any of the three circuit configurations from outside the body, by means of the magnetic switch.

The advantage of the *P* wave synchronous mode is that the heart is paced by the SA node activity, and it therefore changes rate according to metabolic demand. Its use would be indicated by AV node disease, for example.

The invention of the microprocessor chip in the 1970s meant that pacemaker signal processing could be done by an implanted computer. This has introduced extensive flexibility among the features that can be programmed into an implantable pacemaker. With the microprocessor, it is possible to store the patient's ECG distinctive features in memory and calculate parameters such as the *P–R* interval, *QRS* duration, and *S–T* interval. On the basis of this data, the pacing stimulus could then be chosen by the pacemaker. The microprocessor therefore introduces considerable complexity into the pacemaker. Choosing the proper mode of operation likewise becomes complicated, requiring a knowledge of both pacemaker capabilities and medical practice. A programmable pacemaker is shown in Figure 7.7.

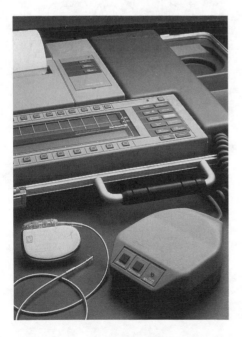

FIGURE 7.7   A programmable pacemaker, lead, and programmer. (Courtesy of Medtronic, Inc.)

PACEMAKER IDENTIFICATION CODE

Pacemakers are designed to stimulate either the atrium or the ventricle of the heart with a stimulating pulse. This stimulus can be controlled or modified by a signal fed back from the heart to the pacemaker. Figure 7.8 shows various configurations of the pacemaker's generator and leads attached to either the right atrium or the right ventricle. The letter *T* on the generator block indicates that a voltage applied there will trigger a stimulus pulse. The letter *I* indicates that a voltage applied there will inhibit the normal stimulus pulsing from the stimulus-pulse generator. In more complex pacemakers, the feedback lead will interrogate a logic circuit as part of a microprocessor.

The available configurations of the pacemaker are given by a five-letter code established by the North American Society of Pacing and

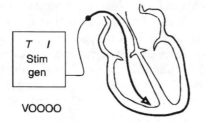
(a)

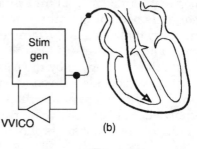
(b)

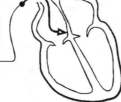
(c)

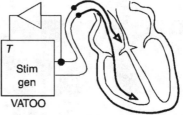
(d)

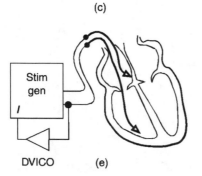
(e)

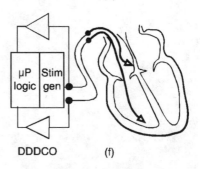
(f)

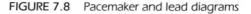

FIGURE 7.8 Pacemaker and lead diagrams

Electrophysiology and the British Pacing and Electrophysiology Group, jointly referred to as NBG. The five-letter code is given in Table 7.1 (see Teplitz, pp. 1–8). A similar code is published by the American Society for the Advancement of Medical Instrumentation. It is important to note that all pacing modes are not completely described by the code; it is necessary to read the manufacturer's literature for a complete description.

Letter one of the code identifies which chamber of the heart is paced—either the right ventricle or the right atrium. D means that both chambers are paced, and 0 means that neither chamber is paced. *Letter two* of the code identifies the chamber from which voltages used to control the pacemaker are sensed. *Letter three* identifies the manner in which the stimulus sensed from the heart controls the pacemaker. The sensed voltage either triggers (or fires) the pacemaker or inhibits the pacemaker from delivering a pulse (turns it off). It may do both, depending on the timing. *Letter four* of the code identifies the various features the pacemaker may have. The *fifth letter* of the code identifies pacemakers that are capable of treating tachycardia.

TABLE 7.1   Pacemaker Identification Code

LETTER ONE—CHAMBER(S) PACED
  A—Atrium
  V—Ventricle
  D—Dual (both chambers)
  O—None
LETTER TWO—CHAMBER(S) SENSED
  A—Atrium
  V—Ventricle
  D—Dual
  O—None
LETTER THREE—RESPONSE MODE
  T—Triggered
  I—Inhibited
  O—No response
  D—Dual
LETTER FOUR—PROGRAMMABLE FUNCTIONS
  P—Programmable (rate and/or output only)
  M—Multiprogrammable
  C—Communicating (noninvasive programmable)
  O—Nonprogrammable
  R—Rate modulation
LETTER FIVE—TACHYARRHYTHMIA FUNCTION
  P—Pacing
  S—Shock D
  Dual (P + S)
  O—None

The uses of the code are best illustrated by the examples in Figure 7.8. In part (a), a unipolar pacing lead is implanted into the right ventricle (RV). There is no feedback signal, so an applicable code is VOOOO. Here, the RV is paced at a preset rate that cannot be changed. If the code were VOOPO, it would be possible to change the rate and stimulus level without surgery.

The code in part (b) is VVICO.This means that if the pacemaker senses depolarization activity of the RV (as indicated by the second letter of the code), it will inhibit (as indicated by the third letter) a pacing stimulus to the ventricle (as indicated by the first letter of the code) so that the heart can assume its own rate. This is called a demand pacemaker. The C in the fourth letter position indicates that the stimulus intensity and duration can be changed by programming it with an external unit such as is illustrated in Figure 7.7. The O in the fifth letter position indicates that the pacemaker has no capability in treating tachyarrhythmias.

The code in part (c) indicates preprogrammed pacing of the RA and is coded as AOOOO. In part (d), the code is VATOO. Here, the RA depolarization activity is sensed and fed back to a trigger T on the pacemaker. After an atrioventricular (AV) delay between 150 and 200 ms, the RV is paced. This is the first pacemaker listed that allows the pacing rate to follow metabolic demands. Increases in the SA node rate are followed by the ventricle, and AV synchrony is preserved. This means that, after the appropriate delay, the RV pacing follows the RA depolarization. Asynchrony can result in a 20-percent loss of cardiac output.

The DVICO pacing in part (e) senses the RV and inhibits pacing if the heart is following an adequate sinus rhythm. This introduces demand pacing to conserve battery energy and allow the heart to respond to metabolic demands. It also preserves AV synchrony by pacing first the RA then the RV after the appropriate interval.

The modes for pacing were developed sequentially to deal with problems that arose in the clinic, culminating with DDDCO pacing, which is illustrated in part (f) of Figure 7.8. This pacing has the fewest drawbacks, unless added complexity is considered a drawback. It can be programmed in several modes of operation, including atrial and ventricular sensing (which indicate that the normal sinus rhythm exists), ventricular pacing with atrial sensing, atrial pacing with ventricular sensing, and a combination of atrial and ventricular pacing.

Rate Modulation

When disease prevents the heart rate from responding to metabolic demand, rate-sensitive pacemakers can be used. Such devices have been developed to sense the need for heart rate changes in order to maintain a cardiac output sufficient to satisfy increased metabolic demand due to exercise or parasympathetic responses (see Fabiszewski).

One activity sensor consists of a piezoelectric crystal bonded to the pulse generator case. Certain types of exercise cause increased vibration of the casing, which stimulates a crystal that in turn signals the pacemaker to speed up. The advantage of the device is that it is simple and does not require added sensors on the heart. The rate, however, may not exactly follow demand, as in the case of smooth action exercise such as biking and swimming. On the other hand, a rough-riding vehicle could make the heart rate go up when there was not a sufficient metabolic demand to justify it.

A second sensor measures RV blood temperature, which increases after sustained exercise. The rate control sensor responds to exercise, but not to the emotions.

A third rate control mechanism measures the transthoracic electrical impedance, which follows the breathing rate and tidal volume. An increased breathing rate would thereby stimulate an increased heart rate as well. The advantage of the mechanism is that it uses conventional implanted leads and correlates well the metabolic need in patients with normal respiratory function. Abnormal respiratory function, however, may be a contraindication for its use.

A fourth mechanism results from the fact that the Q–T interval of the ECG shortens with increased exercise. In addition to physical metabolic demands, Q–T sensing pacemakers respond to mental metabolic demands and control the pacing rate accordingly.

INDICATIONS FOR PACEMAKER USE

The pacemaker is indicated for use when there is disease of the SA node, the atrium, AV node, or of the ventricle of the heart. That is, cardiac pacing is indicated when there is a significant problem with the heart's electrical conduction system.

These conduction problems are manifested as delays, blocks, reentrant tachyarrhythmias, and other malfunctions in the electrical system that may lead to a decrease in cardiac output. Symptoms such as syncope, vertigo, palpitations, shortness of breath, chest tightness, confusion, exercise intolerance, and congestive heart failure may result.

If AV conduction is intact but a sick sinus syndrome (SSS) occurs, the physician may order AAICO pacing. This paces the RA unless sensed activity there inhibits the pacemaker. This would treat bradycardia. If, in addition, there was chronotropic incompetence, rate modulation may be ordered as AAIRO pacing. A complete or partial AV block may be treated with VVICO. Again, the addition of chronotropic incompetence would require VVIRO pacing so that pacing could respond to metabolic demands. Dual chamber pacing is indicated for patients who have an AV block. Patients with SSS and AV block may require DVICO pacing.

It may be programmed to inhibit both RA and RV pacing if a normal activity is sensed in both chambers, as may be the case in second-degree heart block in which the heart is only intermittently blocked.

In the case of a tachydysrhythmia, a DDDCP mode may be indicated. This may be programmed so that when tachycardia is sensed, a faster stimulus is delivered to the pacing lead at the proper time to overdrive the reentrant circuit and terminate the tachycardia. In one tachycardia-treating pacemaker the treatment consists of a pacing pulse train having a time period less than the detected ventricular tachycardia (VT). This "burst" of pacing pulses is repeated up to 15 times at progressively shorter periods between the pulses, in order to terminate the VT (see Zacouto). These are pacing pulses, requiring very little energy from the battery, and do not shorten the battery lifetime the way a defibrillating shock would. Clearly, the introduction of the microprocessor into the pacemaker has given the physician such flexibility in treatment that a detailed study of not only heart disease but the pacemaker also needs to be made before competent prescriptions can be made. Both of these in-depth studies are beyond the scope of this book.

CONTRAINDICATIONS FOR PACEMAKER USE

Permanent cardiac pacing is contraindicated when medications are effective in treating ECG abnormalities. It is contraindicated when the SA node and AV conduction paths are only transiently interrupted due to an acute myocardial infarction. Dual chamber pacing is not indicated to treat atrial fibrillation because of the lack of a reliable RA depolarization to trigger RV pacing. Dual pacing may not be indicated for those with physically small hearts in whom electrode cross talk (induced signal coupling between pacemaker leads) can be especially troublesome. Pacemaker implantation is also contraindicated in patients with active infections. These patients should be treated with antibiotics and temporary pacing until the infection is resolved.

PERMANENT PACEMAKER INSERTION AND POSTOPERATIVE CARE

Permanent pacemaker implantation is performed by the surgeon in a sterile environment where all of the necessary equipment is available. The procedure is usually done with the patient under local anesthesia. The pacing lead system is inserted (transvenously) via a vein (subclavian, cephalic, or external or internal jugular) into the apex of the right ventricle. The pulse generator is placed in a small subcutaneous pocket inferior to the clavicle.

Immediate postoperative nursing care includes monitoring the patient's vital signs until he or she is stable. It is important to rule out pneumothorax, the collapse of the lung on the affected side caused by air or gas in the pleural cavity due to a punctured lung. Pneumothorax can occur as a complication of obtaining venous access during permanent pacemaker insertion. It is also important to confirm proper electrode position, and secure a baseline for future clinical evaluations with an anterior–posterior (AP) and lateral chest X ray and a baseline ECG. The patient should be evaluated for an adequate cardiac output with the current pacing mode. During pacing, assess skin color and temperature, syncope, mental status changes, and blood pressure. For at least 48 hours, the patient must be taught not to move the affected arm and shoulder vigorously, because this can increase incisional pain or dislodge the pacemaker lead.

Patients should be thoroughly reevaluated two to four weeks after pacemaker insertion. The post-insertion history should document a relief of all pre-pacer symptoms. The physical examination should be performed with attention to the insertion site and pacemaker pocket. Pacemaker function should be assessed with the use of a magnet and ECG monitoring. Recognition of abnormal pacemaker function requires a complete understanding of normal function. It may be difficult to recognize what a certain patient's normal pacer function is because many different types of implanted pacemakers exist. Therefore, it is important to teach the patient to carry a card that identifies the pacemaker manufacturer, model and serial number, pacing mode, date of implantation, current medications, and other pertinent information. Later follow-up includes a combination of office or clinic visits and trans-telephonic monitoring.

Important teaching includes showing the patient how to take his or her own pulse daily. If the pulse rate is not within the acceptable limit, the patient should be instructed to call a physician. The nurse should stress the importance of having the patient report the return of any symptoms of hemodynamic instability, such as chest pain, dizziness, palpitations, shortness of breath, and peripheral edema, seen prior to pacer insertion. The return of these symptoms may signal inadequate pacemaker settings and warrant a reprogramming of the pacemaker. Also, the nurse should teach the patient to be aware of potential early and late complications of pacemaker use, as described in the following section.

COMPLICATIONS OF PERMANENT PACEMAKER USE

Complications of pacemaker use can be classified as difficulties associated with the insertion procedure, the maintenance of an intravascular and intracardiac foreign body, and the pacing hardware itself.

The complications associated with the insertion procedure include venous thrombosis, embolism, pneumothorax, arterial trauma, arrhythmias induced by pacemaker insertion, inappropriate lead placement resulting in chest wall or diaphragmatic pacing, and myocardial perforation leading to cardiac tamponade.

Significant thrombosis of the veins used for pacemaker lead insertion is a rare complication. Pulmonary embolism due to thrombus on the pacing wire is also very rare. Anticoagulation and thrombolytic therapy are generally effective treatment measures. Thrombectomy should be considered if a large intracardiac thrombus is diagnosed.

A perforated ventricle may occur if the pacing lead passes through the heart into the pericardial sac. This displaced lead may pace the chest wall or diaphragm, resulting in uncomfortable skeletal muscle contractions and a failure to pace on the ECG.

Watch for these signs and symptoms of a perforated ventricle with resultant cardiac tamponade: distant heart sounds, hypotension, pulsus paradoxus, narrowed pulse pressure, distended neck veins, cyanosis, restlessness, or decreased urine output.

Complications due to the maintenance of an intravascular and intracardiac foreign body include infection of the pacemaker leads and pulse generator. Like any foreign body, the pacemaker leads and generator may result in vague symptoms, such as increased WBCs or temperature, which may lead to sepsis. Infections associated with the pacemaker generator are more common early after pacemaker insertion and may be due to improper incision care.

The incision site should be kept clean and dry until it heals, which is usually in seven to ten days. Clothing should be worn loosely around the generator site, because tight clothes may irritate the site and lead to infection. Symptoms of generator site infection include redness, warmth, swelling, and exudate at the insertion site. Therapy should include aspiration, culture, and drainage of the pus. Although treatment almost always requires removal of the pacing system, antibiotics should be tried first. Prophylactic antibiotics should be used when undergoing invasive dental procedures.

Complications can also occur with the pacing system and can include loss of pacing and sensing capabilities, pacemaker induced arrhythmias, generator malfunction or failure, electromagnetic interference from the outside, or an inappropriate response to programming.

A summary of these complications is given in Table 7.2.

Pacemaker Failures

In a small number of patients, early failure to sense or capture may occur due to catheter dislodgement. Increasing the sensitivity or output

TABLE 7.2   Permanent Pacemaker Complications

Insertion Procedure
  Venous thrombosis
  Embolism
  Hemothorax, pneumothorax
  Arterial trauma
  Arrhythmias
  Chest wall or diaphragm pacing
  Cardiac tamponade

Maintenance of a Foreign Body
  Infection of the leads
  Infection of the pulse generator

Pacing Hardware
  Loss of pacing
  Loss of sensing
  Pacemaker induced arrhythmias
  Generator malfunction or failure
  Outside electromagnetic interference
  Inappropriate response to programming

amplitude may remedy the situation. If reprogramming is unsuccessful, early reparation with repositioning is indicated.

After an endocardial lead has been placed, fibrosis will gradually occur around the tip. The fibrosis allows the lead tip to adhere to the myocardium. This fibrosis may contribute to a gradual increase in stimulus threshold as well as a decreased ability to sense. Myocardial infarction may lead to an increased threshold and a failure to capture. Oversensing may send a false inhibit signal to the pacemaker and allow a bradycardia to persist. Also, a failure to capture may result in bradycardia and lead to ischemia and chest pain. Therefore, pacemaker malfunctions may be a result of or a cause of myocardial ischemia. Increasing the sensitivity or output stimulus amplitude may correct the problem.

Lead disconnection or fracture may occur after a period of time due to stress at the lead connection site to the generator. It may also occur from blunt chest trauma, where the lead is torn away from the generator. Diagnosis of lead disconnection or fracture can be made by a chest radiograph.

Battery failure may result in either failure to sense or pace. Newer pacemakers exhibit a gradual slowing of the pacing rate as the battery fails. Even though newer batteries last for years, the patient should keep track of his or her pulse daily and immediately report any discrepancies with the programmed rate.

Late complications include a reoccurrence of the original symptoms; electrode or wire fracture, displacement, or perforation of the heart or vessels; infection; deep venous thrombosis; pacemaker related tachycardias; premature generator failure; myoinhibition; chest wall pacing; diaphragmatic pacing; and electromagnetic interference from the outside.

The loss of sensing may require a sensitivity adjustment. The loss of pacing or the failure to capture may require an increase of stimulus intensity or duration or a check of the electrode position with X ray. Infection may be indicated by redness of the skin or increased temperature. Bradycardia or tachycardia is indicated by pulse rate or the ECG waveform. The ECG will show the stimulus pulse from the pacemaker before the *P* wave or the *QRS* complex, or both as appropriate. Inspection of the ECG will give evidence of pacing generator malfunctions. Although much progress has been made in shielding the pacemaker, strong radiations, such as those from an electrosurgical unit (ESU), a magnetic resonance imager (MRI) or security systems, should be avoided. The patient who feels an interference should be instructed to walk away from the source of it. A summary of symptoms and pacemaker failures is given in Table 7.3.

STERILIZATION

Most pacemakers are delivered by the manufacturer in sterile packages that should be opened in sterile areas for immediate implantation.

Because of the batteries, most pacemakers cannot be sterilized by steam autoclave, which requires exposure to 121° C for 20 to 30 minutes. Therefore, the principle means of sterilization by the manufacturer is by ethylene oxide (ETO) sterilization, which operates at 57° C. ETO is highly toxic, and ambient exposure to personnel must be limited to 2 parts per million (ppm), according to Occupational Safety and Health Administration (OSHA) regulations. To eliminate residue on the implant, the device is aerated for seven days before use. Also, after packaging, X-ray radiation sterilization is used.

In mass production, it is economical to use radiation sterilization by X ray; however, the capital cost of the equipment cannot be justified in many hospital situations.

PACEMAKER REUSE

Some pacemakers may be implanted in a patient for a very short time and removed because of a change in the prescribed therapy or the death of the patient. Because they are expensive, it is cost effective to reuse them. But because of the problems with sterilization just mentioned, this may be difficult to do in the hospital. The manufacturer, however, should be able to perform this task.

TABLE 7.3   Symptoms and Hardware Failures

FAILURE TO PACE

Generator
   Battery failure
   Maladjustment of stimulus or sensing levels

Lead faults
   Fracture or disconnection from the unit or heart

ECG recording difficulty
   Lead fault
   Inadequate gain setting

Internal inhibition
   Appropriate sensing of faster intrinsic rate
   Inappropriate oversensing

External inhibition
   Sensing of electrical interference

FAILURE TO CAPTURE

Generator
   Battery failure

Lead faults
   Displacement, disconnection, fracture, or perforation

Threshold change
   Increase with time
   Fibrosis of tip
   Acute MI

Drugs
   Electrolyte abnormalities

FAILURE TO SENSE

Generator
   Battery failure
   Maladjustment of sensing or stimulus levels

Lead faults
   Displacement, fracture, or perforation
   Fibrosis around tip

Electrical Interference

Decreased *QRS* amplitude
   Acute MI
   Drugs
   Metabolic changes

TEMPORARY PACING

Indications for temporary pacing are summarized in Table 7.4. When symptomatic SA node dysfunction occurs, and cardioactive medications are ineffective, a temporary pacemaker may be needed to restore an effective heart rate. Temporary pacing is also effective for high-degree AV block and slow ventricular escape rhythms.

Temporary pacing is also indicated for the termination of various atrial and ventricular tachyarrhythmias. Overdrive pacing has been successfully used to terminate reentrant arrhythmias involving the SA node, AV node, and the ventricles. Pacing can also be used to suppress several tachyarrhythmias. Pacing at a faster rate than the tachycardia can inhibit the reentrant pulse causing the tachyarrhythmia.

During an acute MI, hemodynamically unstable rhythms that are either present or likely to occur necessitate temporary pacing. These rhythms include certain types of AV conduction abnormalities and bundle blocks. For example, temporary pacing is used for Type II AV block associated with the anterior MI since it may progress to complete AV block.

Prophylactic temporary pacing is indicated in situations that may result in a hemodynamically unstable patient. These settings include those during acute MI, those after cardiac surgery, those during right heart catheterization in patients with left bundle branch block, and those with therapeutic administration of drugs that produce bradycardia.

TABLE 7.4   Indications for Temporary Pacing

Symptomatic Bradyarrhythmias
   Sick sinus syndrome
   Complete heart block
   Bradycardia

Tachyarrhythmias
   Atrial flutter
   Torsades de pointes ventricular tachycardia
   Tachycardia

During Acute Myocardial Infarction (MI)
   Symptomatic bradycardia
   Type II second-degree AV block
   Third-degree AV block
   New bifasicular block
   New left or right bundle branch block (LBBB or RBBB) with anterior MI

Prophylactic Pacing
   Mobitz II second-degree AV block
   After cardiac surgery
   Right heart catheterization with LBBB

Emergency Invasive Pacing

Emergency pacing takes place when the heart must be paced temporarily, and implantation is not indicated. The pacing may be done either *invasively* by inserting a catheter into the heart through the skin. Or it may be done *non-invasively* by applying the stimulus to the surface of the skin, and allowing the currents to flow into the heart. (See Martinez.)

Emergency pacing may be indicated for patients with bradydysrhythmias, SSS, the Stokes-Adams syndrome (an altered state of consciousness caused by a decrease in blood flow to the brain), and Torsades de pointes (a very rapid ventricular tachycardia characterized by a gradually changing *QRS* complex in the ECG). Emergency pacing is used to prevent progressive heart block from a myocardial infarction and, in case of an implanted pacemaker, failure.

An external temporary pacemaker, such as the one illustrated in Figure 7.9, may be used for emergency pacing. Before inserting the pacemaker, the procedure should be explained to the patient. Sedation should also be given to alleviate the local discomfort the patient will feel at the insertion site. An IV line should be established for the possible administration of emergency drugs, in case ventricular arrhythmia is caused by the insertion procedure. A physician may choose to

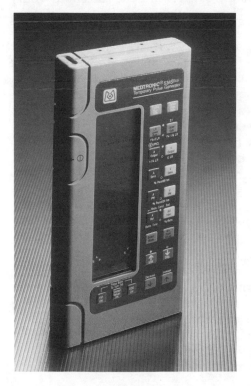

FIGURE 7.9   An external pacemaker (Courtesy of Medtronic, Inc.)

use a subclavian and internal jugular vein to insert the pacing catheter. A balloon-tipped and bipolar semirigid pacing catheter may be guided by fluoroscopic monitoring. The catheter is inserted under ECG control. As the catheter enters the RA, *P* waves become prominent on the ECG. As it enters the RV, the *QRS* amplitude increases. The *QRS* will decrease if the tip goes too far into the pulmonary artery.

Once the catheter is in place, it should be sutured and the insertion site should be dressed using sterile technique. If a femoral or brachial approach is used, immobilize the extremity to avoid pulling at the pacing wires.

Initially, both the ventricle output and sensitivity are set to the minimum. The emergency physician chooses a pacing rate, perhaps 70 bpm. After the lead is placed in the ventricle terminal of the pacemaker, the ventricle output pulse is increased until one-to-one capture of the *QRS* is achieved. This is indicated by a pacing artifact immediately preceding the *QRS* on the ECG. The ventricle sensitivity will then be increased by the physician until the pacemaker inhibits the pacing pulse, when the demand mode is desired and achievable.

The pacemaker threshold (the minimum amount of current that will stimulate a paced heartbeat) should be checked every shift or as ordered and documented in the nurses' notes. Check the hospital protocol before measuring the threshold. To determine the threshold, verify one-to-one capture on the ECG. Then gradually decrease the milliamps until a wide *QRS* complex is no longer seen after the pacemaker spike. This means that one-to-one capture is lost. If the patient's intrinsic rhythm is greater than the rate set on the pacemaker, and is overriding the pacemaker, increase the pacemaker rate to about 10 bpm above the patient's rate to obtain a paced rhythm. Next, increase the milliamps slowly to find the point at which capture is again achieved. This is the pacing threshold. Set the ventricular output at two to three times this threshold to allow a safety margin. Be careful not to overstimulate the heart, as this could cause VT or VF.

The sensitivity threshold (the number of millivolts needed to inhibit the pacemaker from firing) should also be checked as per hospital policy and documented in the nurses' notes. When the heart voltage feedback exceeds the threshold, the pacemaker will be inhibited from firing. If the pacemaker is set in the asynchronous mode, it will ignore the feedback and pace at its own fixed rate.

To check the sensitivity threshold, set the pacer rate at least 10 bpm less than the patient's intrinsic rate. Decrease the sensitivity to the most sensitive position (approximately 1.5 mV). Ensure that the output is set high enough to cause capture. At these settings, the pacemaker should begin sensing the feedback and be inhibited from firing. On some pacemakers, sensing will be indicated by a flashing light. Next, slowly decrease the pacemaker's sensitivity (i.e., increase the voltage feedback requirement) until the pacemaker ceases sensing and begins firing. Turn the sensitivity up until sensing occurs again; this is the sensitivity threshold. Reset the sensitivity so that it is two or three times more sensitive than the threshold.

Careful adjustment of the pacemaker parameters requires skill, experience, and appropriate certification. Once the parameters are set and checked, a protective mechanism is used to prevent tampering.

Complications

In addition to the complications mentioned with permanent pacing, temporary pacing carries its own risks, such as microshock. In temporary pacing, the pacemaker wires may be exposed. This makes the patient vulnerable to the microshock (see Chapters 1 and 2). This means that only 10 µA of current will put the patient at risk of a ventricular fibrillation (VF). When not in the pacemaker, the leads should be covered with a dry insulator, such as a gauze pad, to insulate them from the patient and everything else in the environment. Any attendant who touches the leads should take precautions against mediating leakage current from such objects as the bed, monitoring equipment, and lamps, or coupling to electromagnetic waves in the environment. Insulating gloves must be worn by anyone touching the leads, and the person needs to be grounded with the patient to dispel any electrostatic charge. One way to do this is to have the patient hold your bare arm with his or her bare hand before you touch the catheter. The patient must be carefully monitored for VF, and a defibrillator and a qualified operator needs to be present. This precaution is also necessary if the setting of the pacemaker dials needs to be changed for any reason.

Symptoms of Pacemaker Malfunction

Symptoms of pacemaker malfunction are listed in Table 7.5. These symptoms may be indicated by a change in the patient's mental status, low blood pressure, or an abnormal cardiac rhythm, including bradycardia, tachycardia, or premature ventricular contractions. A change in skin color or skin temperature or low urine output can be caused by a faulty pacemaker. The presence of crackles in the lung sounds that do not clear with coughing may indicate cardiac tamponade secondary to a perforated ventricle. Any of the situations listed under the section "Complications of Permanent Pacemaker Use" apply as well.

To be able to identify the type of pacemaker malfunction that is occurring, one must be able to interpret rhythms on an ECG. The ECG is discussed more fully in Chapter 4. Figure 7.10(a) shows a properly functioning pacemaker where a wide *QRS* complex follows the pacing

TABLE 7.5　Symptoms of Temporary Pacemaker Malfunction

FAILURE TO PACE

Possible problem:
　　Dislodged catheter
　　Loose catheter terminals
　　Broken catheter wires
　　Battery/generator failure
　　Pacemaker turned off
　　Sensing or pacing maladjustment

FAILURE TO CAPTURE

Possible problem:
　　Dislodged catheter
　　Fracture lead
　　Increased threshold
　　Battery failure
　　Maladjustment

FAILURE TO SENSE

Possible problem:
　　Dislodged catheter
　　Pacemaker on asynchronous mode
　　Competition between patient and pacemaker rates
　　Increased sensing threshold
　　Maladjustment

spike. If the sensitivity control is properly adjusted, there may be no demand for the pacing pulse, and it will be absent from a normal ECG trace. Part (b) of the figure illustrates the ECG that results when the pacer does not capture the heart. Here, a pacing spike is not followed by a *QRS* complex. This may be caused by a low ventricular output setting from the pacemaker. The electrode connection to the heart may increase in resistance or become dislodged. A chest X ray may be used to check the position of the electrode. Interventions include turning the patient on the left side to aid electrode contact with the myocardium, increasing the ventricular output, replacing the battery, or having the physician replace the fractured lead.

In part (c), the pacemaker is undersensing and does not inhibit the pacing pulse. At the same time, the pacing spike does not capture the heart. This may result in a pacing signal that occurs during the *T* wave when the heart is vulnerable to fibrillation, and a pacemaker induced VF could occur. To intervene, turn the sensitivity dial to a more sensi-

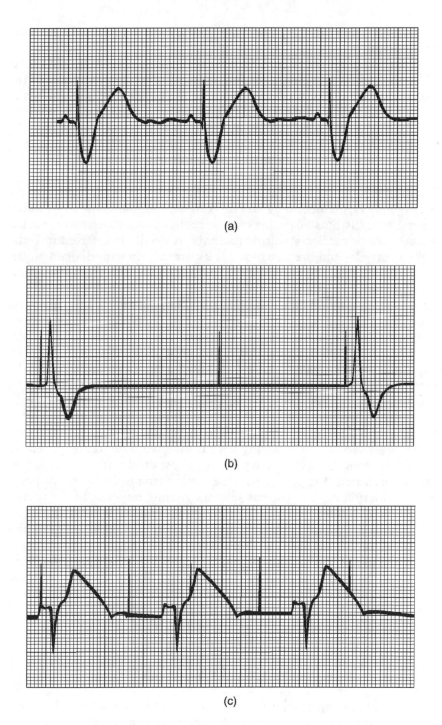

(a)

(b)

(c)

FIGURE 7.10   Packing spikes in the ECG

tive position and call the physician to reposition or replace the catheter immediately.

If the pacer is not pacing, make sure the pacemaker is turned on, replace the battery and generator, and tighten the connection between the pacemaker generator and leads. Monitor the patient's vital signs while calling a physician immediately. Prepare to insert new leads or attempt to pace the patient with another mode, such as transcutaneous pacing.

Transthoracic Pacing

When time is limited and no other technique is available, transthoracic pacing may be performed by an emergency physician. Due to its quick insertion, transthoracic pacing may be preferable to transvenous pacing in unstable or cardiac-arresting patients. A needle is inserted into the right ventricle, and the free blood is aspirated. An experienced physician can position the needle in 30 to 45 seconds, therefore interrupting CPR only briefly. The pacing wire is then introduced, and the needle is removed. A temporary pacemaker is connected to this wire. Emergency pacing is instituted with the same settings used for temporary transvenous pacing.

Nursing responsibilities during insertion are similar to those when a transvenous pacemaker is inserted. The nurse must be monitoring the patient's vital signs and response procedure. As the pacing wire enters the ventricle, venous access and antiarrhythmic drugs should be available to treat any ventricular arrhythmias. A functioning pacing generator must be available for attachment to the pacing wire. All connections must be secured after the pacing wire is inserted. The pacing generator should be securely taped to the patient's chest until transvenous pacing can be instituted. The patient's ECG should then display adequate pacemaker functioning. The patient's hemodynamic response to the pacing should be monitored carefully. Finally, the pacemaker settings should be documented. The same care should be taken regarding the patient's electrical safety as is taken with transvenous pacing.

Because of the serious potential complications, this procedure must only be used in the most dire situations. Potential complications include pericardial tamponade, coronary artery laceration, conduction system damage, puncture of mediastinal or abdominal organs, and pneumothorax (a collection of air in the pleural cavity).

NONINVASIVE PACING

Noninvasive pacing has the advantage of not requiring a central venous catheter with all its risks of infection and vessel and organ perforation. Noninvasive pacing may be indicated for acute myocardial infarction, heart block, a temporary arrhythmia, asystole after administration of epinephrine and atropine, the transport of cardiac patients, or as a temporary measure until another pacing form can be administered.

Transcutaneous Pacing

The popularity of noninvasive transcutaneous pacing (NTP) has been greatly increased due to such recent improvements as decreased patient discomfort, the ability to pace in the demand mode, and the reduction in interference at the central monitor. NTP has many advantages over temporary transvenous pacing. These advantages include the quick and easy initiation of pacing. The administration of pacing can occur in the emergency room or in the patient's hospital room; it can even occur prehospital, by a variety of health-care professionals, with patient stabilization occurring within one to two minutes. The American Heart Association has even included the use of NTP as an intervention in the algorithm for symptomatic bradycardia.

Transcutaneous pacing is administered through gelled adhesive electrodes approximately 7 to 10 cm in diameter. A posterior electrode is placed on the back below the scapula and to the left of the spine. The anterior electrode is placed on the left side of the precordium (overlying the heart). On a female, it is important to avoid placing this electrode over breast tissue, because this may increase discomfort. It is important that the diaphragm not be mistakenly paced because the electrode is placed too low. This will result in dyspnea.

The skin is prepared by clipping excess hair, but not shaving or abrading the skin. This could cause high-current regions and burns in the razor nicks. Either pre-gelled or conductive adhesive electrodes may be used. If pre-gelled electrodes are used, make sure they are moist. If metal electrodes are used, take care not to allow the gel to exceed the electrode diameter; this will cause stray current paths. ECG electrodes are also placed so that the ECG can be monitored during the pacing procedure.

To capture the heartbeat, a pacemaker rate greater than the observed heart rate is chosen. The pacemaker applies a pacing pulse between 5 and 40 ms in duration.

These external pacemakers have the capacity to function in the demand mode. Pacing rates range from 30 to 180 bpm. The output in milliamperes ranges from 0 to 200 mA, with the average mA range needed to capture the myocardium being 60 to 80 mA. Pulse width (or stimulus duration) usually ranges from 20 to 40 ms, enabling the pacemaker to capture the myocardium at a lower mA for longer durations and possibly decreasing patient discomfort.

To implement transcutaneous pacing, apply the electrodes and set the pacing above the patient's intrinsic rate. Begin with the mA at 0 and increase slowly until capture is obtained. During an arrest situation, apply the electrodes and set the desired heart rate. Begin with the mA at 60. If capture does not occur, gradually increase the mA until capture is reached.

Complications

Complications that are commonly seen with transcutaneous pacing include painful stimulation, failure to sense from the ECG, and failure to capture. Patients can experience pain from the contraction of the chest wall muscle during pacing. Patient discomfort is reduced if the stimulation is below 55 mA. Proper electrode positioning and proper adherence to the skin will decrease the mA needed for pacing. If the patient is still uncomfortable, pain medication may be helpful.

Failure to sense the intrinsic *QRS* will cause the pacemaker to pace inappropriately. This inability to sense can occur when the ECG electrodes become detached. Therefore, the adherence of the ECG electrodes should be monitored frequently and replaced as needed, especially with restless or diaphoretic patients. Remember to turn the pacemaker to the "monitor only" mode when changing the electrodes, so inappropriate pacing does not occur.

Failure to capture may also occur due to poor electrode contact. Subtle changes in the patient's condition, such as electrolyte imbalances, ischemia, or new drug therapies, may increase the pacing threshold. Because the NTP's mA level is set only 5 to 10 mA above the pacing threshold to minimize patient discomfort, frequent changes in the mA may be needed to maintain capture. The heart can be driven into tachycardia or ventricular fibrillation. Therefore, a defibrillator, often built into the temporary pacer, should be present. Appropriate medication to treat arrythmias should also be available.

TRANSCUTANEOUS ELECTRICAL NERVE STIMULATION

Transcutaneous electrical nerve stimulation (TENS) was introduced in the early 1970s by P. Wall, W. H. Sweet, and R. Melzack. A TENS unit consists of a pulse generator driving two electrodes that are placed on the skin near a source of pain, such as a surgical incision, as shown in Figure 7.11. Serving as an analgetic, its purpose is to relieve pain.

There are two types of pain. *Acute pain* results from the stimulation of a pain receptor due to injury, pressure, chemical stimulus, heat, cold, or electrical current. Acute pain is relieved after the stimulus that causes it is removed or inhibited. *Chronic pain* persists even after the

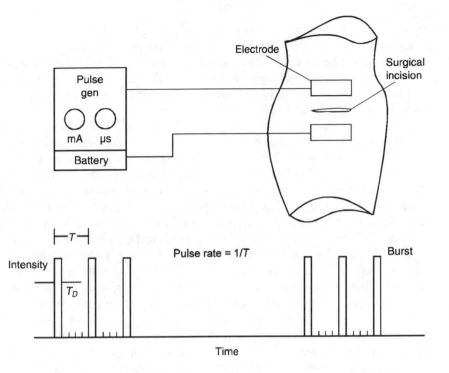

FIGURE 7.11   A TENS unit

original source of the pain has been removed for a long period of time. For example, pain may be felt from a phantom limb after an amputation.

To understand how the TENS unit functions to relieve pain, one must have an understanding of the gate control theory of pain. This theory proposes that a gate which exists in the spinal cord is opened or closed by certain afferent nerve fibers selectively allowing impulses regarding sensation and pain to reach the brain. Different classes (A, B, and C) of afferent nerve fibers exist on the skin's surface. These fibers carry information regarding sensation to the brain. Of these fibers, there are two that carry information regarding pain. These nerve endings are either the rapidly conducting myelinated A delta fibers or the slower unmyelinated C fibers. The skin also has receptors attached to large-diameter nerve fibers, the activation of which may decrease or eliminate pain. Therefore, it is theorized that the TENS unit stimulates the large nerve fibers, which in turn suppress pain stimuli arriving later through the small-diameter slow-conducting fibers at the spinal cord level. This theory is relatively new and still controversial.

The TENS unit produces adjustable pulses of current up to an 80 mA peak value, with a duration of 0 to 500 μS. Peak voltage levels vary up to 500 V. The pulses are delivered at a rate of 1 to 250 Hz. The pulses may be delivered in low-frequency bursts, as illustrated in Figure 7.11. For example, an operator may choose to deliver bursts of seven 100-Hz pulses every 2 seconds for a stimulation period of 30 minutes. In practice, the stimulation settings are generally determined by the individual patient under the guidance of the therapist, and the settings are usually found by trial and error.

The electrodes vary in size from 2 to 6 in^2. They should have sufficient gel or a conductive adhesive, and they should be able to follow the contours of the body. Both reusable and disposable electrodes are available. A gel is used with the reusable electrodes to overcome skin resistance and facilitate electrical current transmission. With proper taping, excellent skin contact can be achieved using reusable electrodes, benefitting the active person. These electrodes need to be washed daily with soap and water. Disadvantages of reusable electrodes include the agility and time required to apply the gel and electrodes. Disposable electrodes are pregelled and possess a self-adhering quality. Many of these electrodes can be used for up to 15 applications, while others are used only once and discarded. Their main advantages are quick and easy application. Unfortunately, they do not adhere as well and tend to fall apart in hot weather. Disposable electrodes should not be washed. The manufacturer should specify the electrode size, and one should not use electrodes specified for another instrument, because the contact resistance may be the wrong value. Most TENS units are battery operated, weigh approximately 130 g, and can be worn on the body.

Indications for Use

TENS has been used for chronic pain for those who suffer the adverse effects of powerful narcotics, such as drug addiction, dizziness, constipation, decrease in mental acuity, and mood changes. Success rates vary from 30 to 70 percent. Success rates as high as 85 percent have been reported when TENS was used in chronic low-back pain.

TENS has also been found effective for phantom limb pain, arthritis, cancer, headaches, and sports related injuries. TENS has even been found particularly effective for relieving acute postoperative pain related to large thoracic and abdominal incisions.

Contraindications for Use

The pulse current of TENS can become as high as an external transcutaneous pacemaker. Therefore, the operator must avoid placing the electrodes so that currents could pass through the heart. For example, one would not use TENS to treat postoperative pain after open-heart surgery except at low, safe current levels. The electrodes should not be placed transcerebally or over delicate structures, such as the larynx, the carotid sinuses, the uterus, or the eyes. High levels of stimulation can cause strong muscle contractions and pain. TENS electrodes should not be placed over sphincters, reflex sites, or other delicate or excitable tissues.

TENS should not be used on some pacemaker patients because the interference may inhibit the pacemaker or cause arrhythmias. In patients with pacemakers, a careful evaluation and extended electrocardiographic monitoring should be performed to ensure that the TENS unit doesn't interfere with the function of the cardiac pacemaker. Most studies involving TENS report either no adverse effects or only minor skin irritation when proper contraindications are observed. TENS should be used only under the direction of a physician or certified health-care provider.

Treatment Procedure

The electrodes should be gelled or have a conductive adhesive. They should be placed on the skin with at least 5 cm between them, as illustrated in Figure 7.12. In postoperative cases, the electrodes are placed on either side of the incision. For chronic low-back pain, they are placed on either side of the lumbar spine. For neck pain, they are placed on either side of the cervical spine. In other cases, the physician may place the electrodes proximal to the painful area. Patients are encouraged to vary electrode positions within the range set by the therapist in order to find the optimal site for pain relief.

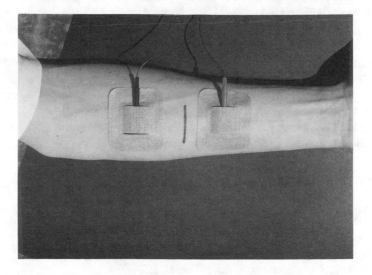

FIGURE 7.12   TENS electrodes relative to a mark that represents an incision.

The pulse intensity may be increased from zero until the patient feels a tingling without muscle contraction. The treatment may last from several minutes to several hours. Patients report a positive relationship between higher intensity TENS and increased analgesia. Thus, it has been seen that patients set TENS stimulation at the highest tolerance level during treatment. Also, there is good evidence that each patient prefers a particular pulse frequency to treat the pain. Therefore, under the direction of a therapist, varied treatments are available for patients to choose.

A second type of treatment is done at a rate of about 2 Hz, using high currents that cause visible muscle contraction. This treatment lasts approximately 30 minutes. In a third type, a brief, intense treatment may be given where the amplitude is set at the highest tolerance level. In many cases, this results in fast relief of pain.

The patient should be instructed to return periodically for follow-up evaluation.

REFERENCES

Allocca, J. A. *Medical Instrumentation for the Health-Care Professional*, Englewood Cliffs, N.J.: Prentice-Hall, Inc., 1991.

Appel-Hardin, S. "The Role of the Critical Nurse in Non-invasive Temporary Pacing." *Critical Care Nurse* 12, no. 13 (1992): 10–19.

Aston, R. *Principles of Biomedical Instrumentation and Measurement*. Riverside, NJ: Macmillan Publishing Co., 1990: Chapter 9.

Bayless, W. "The Elements of Permanent Cardiac Pacing." *Critical Care Nurse* 8, no. 7 (1988): 31–41.

Bocka, J. "External Transcutaneous Pacemakers." *Annals of Emergency Medicine* 18, no. 12 (1989): 1280–86.

Braun, J. "External Transcutaneous Pacemakers." *Annals of Emergency Medicine* 18, no. 12 (1986): 354–59.

Doody, S., et al. "Nonpharmacologic Interventions for Pain Management." *Critical Care Nursing Clinics of North America* 3, no. 1 (1991): 69–75.

Dugan, L. "Permanent Pacemakers." *Nursing91* 21, no. 6 (June 1991): 47–52.

Fabiszewski, R., and K. J. Volosin. "Rate-modulated Pacemakers." *Journal of Cardiovascular Nursing* 5, no. 3 (April 1991): 21–31.

Franklin, J. O., and J. Griffin. "Implantable Devices and Electrotherapy for Arrhythmias." *Hospital Practice* 23, no. 12 (December 15, 1988): 135–50.

Heller, M., et al. "A Comparative Study of Five Transcutaneous Pacing Devices in Unanesthetized Human Volunteers." *Prehospital Disaster Medicine* 4, no 1 (1989): 15–18.

Hickey, C., and L. Baas. "Temporary Cardiac Pacing." *AACN Clinical Issues in Critical Care Nursing* 2, no. 1, (1991): 107–17.

Johnson, M. et al. "An In-depth Study of Long-term Users of TENS: Implications for Clinical Use." *Pain* 44 (1991): 221–29.

Kinney, M., et al. *AACN's Clinical Reference for Critical Care Nursing*. New York: McGraw-Hill, 1988: 372–97.

Kleinschmidt, K. K., and M. J. Stafford. "Dual-chamber Cardiac Pacemakers." *Journal of Cardiovascular Nursing* 5, no. 3 (April 1991): 9–20.

Martinez, R. "Emergency Cardiac Pacing." *Topics in Emergency Medicine* 10, no. 1 (April 1988): 81–91.

Mund, H., and J. Shuman. "The Indications for Artificial Cardiac Pacemakers." *The Heart*. Edited by J. Hurst. New York: McGraw-Hill, 1990: 561–80.

Owen, A. "Keeping Pace with Temporary Pacing." *Nursing91* 21, no. 4 (April 1991): 58–64.

Pierce, C. "Transcutaneous Cardiac Pacing: Expanding Clinical Applications." *Critical Care Nursing Clinics of North America* 1, no. 2 (1989): 423–35.

Silver, M., and N. Goldschlager. "Temporary Transvenous Cardiac Pacing in the Critical Care Setting." *Chest* 93, no. 3 (1988): 607–13.

Stewart, J., and A. Sheehan. "Permanent Pacemakers: The Nurse's Role in Patient Education and Follow-up Care." *Journal of Cardiovascular Nursing* 5, no. 3 (April 1991): 32–43.

Syverud, S. "Cardiac Pacing." *Emergency Medicine Clinics of North America* 6, no. 2 (1988): 197–215.

Szeto, A. Y. J. "Pain Relief Using Transcutaneous Electrical Nerve Stimulation (TENS)." *Encyclopedia of Medical Devices and Instrumentation*. Vol 4. Edited by J. G. Webster. New York: John Wiley & Sons, 1988: 2203–20.

Teplitz, L. "Transcutaneous Pacemakers." *Journal of Cardiovascular Nursing* 5, no. 3 (April 1991): 44–57.

Teplitz, L. "Classification of Cardiac Pacemakers: The Pacemaker Code." *Journal of Cardiovascular Nursing* 5, no. 3 (April 1991): 1–8.

Textbook of Advanced Cardiac Life Support, 2nd ed. Dallas: American Heart Association, 1990.

Tilkian, A., and E. Daily. *Cardiovascular Procedures*. Washington, D.C.: C.V. Mosby, 1986.

Waggoner, P. "Transcutaneous Cardiac Pacing." *AACN's Clinical Issues in Critical Care Nursing* 2, no. 1 (1991): 118–25.

Welch, T. "Pacemaker Implant: Implications for the Perioperative Nurse." *Association of Operating-room Nurses (AORN) Journal* 49, no. 1 (January 1989): 257–67.

Zacouto, F. I., and L. J. Guize. "Fundamentals of Orthorhythmic Pacing," *Cardiac Pacing Diagnostic and Therapeutic Tools*. Edited by B. Luderitz. New York: Springer-Verlag, 1976: 212–18.

EXERCISES

1. Who was the first person to use a pacemaker in a clinical application?
2. Name a physician who is credited with the first implantable pacemaker.

3. Give the date of the first implantable pacemaker and the name of the design engineer.

4. Who designed the first artificial heart?

5. In whom was the first artificial heart implanted?

6. What is the date of the first implantable pacemaker?

7. What tissue in the heart is its natural pacemaker?

8. What tissue in the heart causes the delay between the contraction of the atrium and the contraction of the ventricle?

9. What is the rate of the ventricle beat when it is self-paced?

10. What is the rate of the sinoatrial node when it is self-paced?

11. Define the following: bradycardia, tachycardia, and asystole.

12. What is the normal range of lead resistances of the pacemaker electrode in contact with the walls of the heart?

13. What factors cause increases in the pacemaker electrode contact resistance?

14. Name the four basic building blocks that are essential to any pacemaker.

15. Draw a block diagram showing the relationship between the three basic building blocks of the pacemaker and the heart, which is being paced in the ventricle.

16. Using Figure 7.3 as a reference, give the stimulation threshold when the pulse duration is 1 ms.

17. Referring to Figure 7.3, if the electrode–heart resistance is 200 ohms, what is the current of the pulse with a duration of 0.5 s?

18. A certain pacemaker paces with a 3 V pulse, 0.25 μs in duration. The heart–electrode resistance is 300 ohms. It has a 2 A-H battery rating. If it paces at 70 bpm, what is the battery lifetime?

19. The pacemaker in exercise 18 is assumed to pace one chamber. If it were operated in the dual chamber mode, what would be the lifetime of the battery?

20. If the pacemaker in exercise 18 were a demand pacemaker that, because of the patient's illness, paced only when he or she slept for 8 hours at night, what would be the battery lifetime?

21. Name three factors that can cause the electrode–heart resistance to increase.

22. Name two types of invasive pacemaker electrode attachments to the heart.

23. What two mechanical features of the endocardial electrode keep it in place in the ventricle?

24. What two mechanical features of the endocardial lead in the atrium keep it in place?

25. If the return path of the current in a pacemaker is through the viscera, what type of electrode does it have.?

26. If the return path of the current in a pacemaker is through an electrode 3 cm displaced on the lead, what type of electrode does it have?

27. Name two methods of compensating for increased electrode–heart resistance.

28. What is the advantage of using a biphasic pulse on the pacemaker?

29. Define the following types of pacemaker:

    Asynchronous

    P-wave synchronous

    R-wave inhibited

    Demand

30. What changes can be made in the stimulus of a VOOPO pacemaker?

31. Which pacemaker, all things being equal except the code, would most likely have a longer battery lifetime, VVICO or VOOCO?

32. Which symptom would the AOORO pacemaker most likely treat, SSS or AV block?

33. Which pacemaker code would be indicated by AV block without any symptom of SSS, AVIOO or VAOOO?

34. Describe two alternative, but equally valid interpretations of a pacemaker code of DDDOO.

35. Define AV synchrony.

36. Which pacemaker code preserves AV synchrony, VVIOO or DVIOO?

37. Name a type of exercise for which a pacemaker that has a rate modulator using a piezoelectric crystal would possibly not increase cardiac output sufficiently.

38. Under what condition might the pacemaker in exercise 37 drive the heart faster than necessary?

39. Under what conditions would temperature feedback not be sufficient to regulate the pacemaker to meet metabolic demand?

40. What two types of feedback mechanisms on a pacemaker would respond to both exercise and emotions in adjusting the rate to meet metabolic demand?

41. Name four regions of the heart that, when diseased, would indicate pacemaker use.

42. If AV conduction is intact but SSS occurs, what pacing mode may be indicated?

43. If AV conduction is impaired, but the atrium is normal, what pacing mode may be indicated?

44. In the case in exercise 43, choose a pacing mode that would not preserve AV synchrony.

45. In the case in exercise 4.3, choose a pacing mode that would preserve AV synchrony and maximize battery lifetime.

46. Describe a pacemaker that would treat tachycardia.

47. Name four contraindications to pacemaker use in patients with heart disease.

48. Name three pacemaker complications involving the blood.

49. Name three electrode and lead related pacemaker complications.

50. Name two early complications that would probably not also appear as late complications to pacemaker use.

51. What sorts of unwanted pacing could occur during pacemaking?

52. What is an indication of low battery power in a pacemaker?

53. Name three symptoms of pacemaker malfunction that can be observed by taking the pulse.

54. Name four symptoms of pacemaker malfunction that can be observed on an ECG display.

55. Redness is seen and heat is felt over the pacemaker. Of what is this symptomatic?

56. The ECG shows pacing pulses that are not in synchrony with any of the ECG distinctive features. What in the pacemaker could cause this?

57. A pacing pulse appears immediately before the *QRS* complex on the ECG, but the *P*-wave is erratic. For what pacing code would this be normal?

58. A pacing spike appears regularly on the ECG display, but there are missing *QRS* complexes. What may be wrong with the pacemaker?

59. Name two types of sterilization used in packaged pacemakers delivered by a manufacturer.

60. Under what conditions is it cost effective to reuse a pacemaker?

61. Name three indications for temporary pacing.

62. Name two indications for permanent pacing that would not also be an indication for emergency pacing.

63. Which is the safer form of emergency invasive pacing if either can be administered under the circumstances: catheter inser-

tion through a jugular vein or transthoracic insertion of the catheter?

64. As the pacemaker lead being inserted into the heart enters the RV, what change occurs in the ECG display taken from that lead?

65. If the pacemaker lead passes into the pulmonary artery, how will this change the ECG display?

66. What complication may result if the pacing pulse is given too high a voltage?

67. What precaution should be taken to protect against microshock when pacemaker wires are exposed?

68. Name two precautions that should be taken by a health-care professional before touching the exposed pacemaker leads.

69. Name four sources of leakage current that could cause a microshock.

70. What changes in the external appearance of a patient are symptoms of possible pacemaker malfunction?

71. What symptoms of pacemaker malfunction may be observed through a stethoscope?

72. What symptoms of pacemaker malfunction are observed on the ECG display?

73. What is the approximate diameter of the electrode used in non-invasive transcutaneous pacing?

74. Give the pacing pulse duration and current level.

75. What precautions must be taken in case transcutaneous pacing causes VT or VF?

76. What is the purpose of TENS?

77. When and by whom was TENS introduced?

78. Define acute pain.

79. Define chronic pain.

80. Draw a block diagram of the TENS unit attached to the forearm of a patient.

81. What is the intensity of the current pulses from a TENS unit?

82. What is the range of TENS pulse duration values?

83. What is the size of the surface electrodes used in TENS?

84. Name four reasons why TENS would be used instead of drugs.

85. Name four conditions that can be treated with TENS.

86. Under what conditions can TENS cause heart arrhythmias?

87. What parts of the anatomy should be avoided when applying TENS?

88. If a patient is treated with TENS for approximately two hours, what should he or she feel and what should the clinician see at the treatment site?

89. If the patient is given a relatively short, intense treatment with TENS, what should the clinician see at the treatment site?

90. Why should TENS be avoided by pacemaker patients?

CHAPTER 8

Lasers and Surgical Devices

From time immemorial, the cold knife has been used in surgery to make incisions, and it is still commonly used. In early times, cautery was done with a hot iron to destroy tissue.

Modern electronic surgical devices were first developed as electrosurgical units (ESUs) by W. T. Bovie in 1924. He used a World War I radio transmitter circuit to make surgical incisions. The second major advance in electronic surgery came with the invention of the laser in 1960 by T. H. Maiman, a Hughes Aircraft Company engineer, who demonstrated laser light from a ruby crystal. By 1965, Polanyi did the first clinical surgery using a CO_2 laser.

The cold knife makes the incision by concentrating the force of the surgeon's hand along a very small cross-sectional area at the sharp blade of the knife. This ruptures the tissue bonds and results in the incision. The electronic surgical devices use one or more of several different principles. They may (1) act as thermal knives and raise the temperature of the cells, causing them to vaporize and part the tissue; (2) have photochemical reactions that break tissue bonds; or (3) have photoplasma that breaks tissue bonds by atomic level impact. The energy of all electronic surgical instruments is absorbed by the tissue and ultimately converted to heat. Unwanted thermal damage to tissue increases with the average power and the duration of contact. Because the laser is capable of using all three processes one cell at a time, it is potentially the most precise of the surgical instruments.

SURGICAL PROCESSES

Specific surgical processes are defined as follows:

Section—To cut tissue.

Incision—Cutting tissue to expose the field of treatment. This may be done with a cold knife, a focused laser, or an ESU using a blade electrode.

185

Excision—Cutting tissue to remove it, using the same tools as for incision.

Coagulation—Using heat to curdle tissue for the purpose of sealing bleeding vessels. This may be done with an ESU that uses a blunt electrode or a pulsed waveform, or with an unfocused laser beam.

Ablation—The removal of a part by excision.

Desiccation—Heating large masses of tissue to dehydrate them and dry them up. This is done with an ESU by inserting an electrode into the tissue.

Fulguration—Causing a spark to fall on tissue, charring it. This is done with a high-voltage ESU needle electrode that is held above the tissue.

LASER SURGICAL DEVICES

The acronym *laser* means "*l*ight *a*mplification by *s*timulated *e*mission of *r*adiation." Lasing of atoms occurs in certain materials when an electron orbiting the atom is raised from its rest state to an excited state by a collision from a pump source. The pump source is either a photon from an external light source or electrons stripped from ions in the vicinity. The excited electron will fall back to its rest state either spontaneously, a rare event, or at will as a result of stimulation from a coherent photon of the same frequency, as illustrated in Figure 8.1. The fall back to the rest state is over a fixed energy gap. The fall results in the emission of a photon of a precise frequency and in phase with the stimulus. Because all of the photons of laser light are in phase with each other, it is called *coherent light*. And because all photons are the same frequency (the same color for visible light), it is called *monochromatic light*. The coherent property of light makes it possible to add

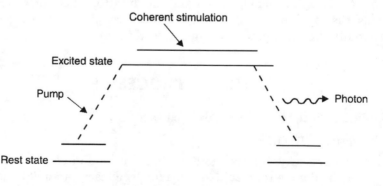

FIGURE 8.1   Lasing

many photons together in a resonator, such as a tube with reflecting mirrors at each end. This amplifies the intensity of the light. The monochromatic property makes it possible to focus laser light into smaller spots than any other kind of light, including sunlight.

GAS TUBE LASER

Lasing for surgery occurs either in a gas, such as CO_2 or argon, or in crystals, such as a yttrium-aluminum-garnet (YAG) alloy. The hardware is rather bulky and inefficient.

In Figure 8.2, which illustrates a gas tube laser, nitrogen and helium are drawn into one chamber of the tube and CO_2 is drawn into another chamber by a vacuum pump. The voltage power supply creates a high current flow and impacts and ionizes the nitrogen, which flows into contact with the CO_2 to act as a lasing pump. The laser light from the CO_2 bounces back and forth between the mirrors at either end of the tube. This resonance builds up the intensity of the light by constructive interference of the light waves. A portion of the light passes through the partially reflective transmitting mirror on the right and emerges as the light output from the laser. The CO_2 laser light has a wavelength of 10.6 microns (10^{-6} meters). For surgical applications, these lasers will typically deliver power levels from 0 to about 100 watts. The lasing process in CO_2 is only about 10 percent efficient. This means that 10 percent of the power appears in the light beam, and the other 90 percent is converted to waste heat. To dissipate it, the cooling system carries the heat away either in water, or another

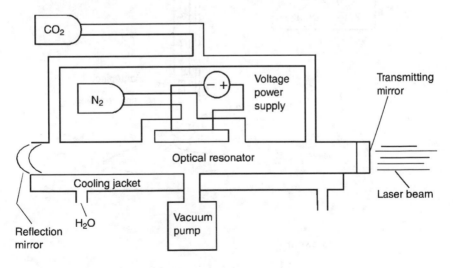

FIGURE 8.2   A CO_2 gas tube laser

suitable fluid. The vacuum pump usually exhausts the contaminated CO_2, although some tubes have closed systems that recycle the gas.

Laser System Optics

To be useful for surgery, the laser light must be directed to the tissue that must be cut, ablated, or desiccated through a flexible arm by means of mirrors, prisms, and lenses. Even more flexibility could be achieved by directing the light through a flexible optical fiber.

CO_2 laser light cannot be passed by the optical fibers currently available, however, and thus must be directed through optical tubing. Also, because the light is not visible, a visible aiming light must be passed through the optics so that the surgeon can use it to focus on the tissue being treated.

In Figure 8.3, the CO_2 laser light is directed toward a turning prism and to a combining mirror. The combining mirror passes the CO_2 light directly through and reflects a portion of the aiming light so that the two light beams travel into the hand piece. The optical lens at the end of the hand piece then focuses both beams on the same spot.

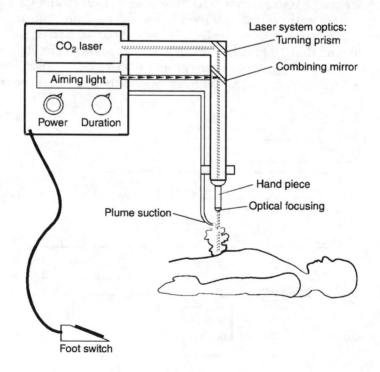

FIGURE 8.3   The CO_2 laser

The surgeon first turns on the aiming light, which may be a low-power helium-neon (He-Ne) laser, to direct the beam to the treatment site. At this low-power level, no significant heating or cutting of the tissue occurs. When the hand piece is accurately aimed, the high-power CO_2 laser light is energized to deliver the treatment.

Just as a musical note has its fundamental pitch, along with overtones, laser light has several modes of vibration. The TM_{00} mode makes a single spot of light in the center of the beam. Because other modes make multiple spots, the CO_2 laser is tuned to the TM_{00} mode. The beam spot can be focused down to a diameter of 0.1 millimeter, which is the size of a living cell.

Spot Size and Power Density

The light from the laser travels in nearly parallel lines and is therefore called *collimated light*. This light enters the hand piece, as illustrated in Figure 8.4, and is brought into focus by the lens at the right end. The spot size on the tissue depends upon the lens position relative to the focal point. The farther away the tissue is from the focal point, the larger will be the spot size on the tissue. A larger spot size produces a smaller power density and causes less of a temperature rise in the tissue. The size of the spot can be adjusted by the focus adjustment if the hand piece is clamped. It can also be adjusted by moving the hand piece relative to the tissue when the hand piece is not clamped.

The power density, P_D, is given by the beam power, P_B, divided by the spot area in the formula

$$P_D = \frac{P_B}{\pi(\frac{d}{2})^2} = 4\,\frac{P_B}{\pi(d)^2} \tag{8.1}$$

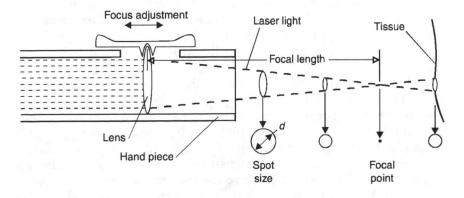

FIGURE 8.4   Optical hand piece

EXAMPLE 8.1   (a) A 100-watt laser produces a spot diameter of 0.1 mm. Calculate the power density. (b) The same laser is defocused to produce a spot diameter of 3 mm to coagulate a bleeding vessel. What is the power density now?

Solution   Equation 8.1 is used to calculate P_D for part (a) as

$$P_D = 4 \frac{100 \text{ W}}{\pi(0.0001 \text{ m})^2}$$
$$= 1.273 \, (10^{10}) \frac{\text{W}}{\text{m}^2}$$

The power density in part (b) is

$$P_D = 4 \frac{100 \text{ W}}{\pi(0.003 \text{ m})^2}$$
$$= 14(10^6) \frac{\text{W}}{\text{m}^2}$$

When you consider that the power density of the sun on the earth is about 1,000 W/m², it is clear from part (a) in Example 8.1 that the laser can expose tissue to 10 million times the heat of the sun as measured on the earth and concentrate it upon a single cell. The result is cell vaporization and tissue incision.

CRYSTAL LASERS

A crystal is a solid with the atoms arranged in an orderly and repetitive form. Many gems such as diamonds and rubies are crystals. In fact, the first laser was made of ruby. A widely used medical laser uses a yttrium-aluminum-garnet (YAG) crystal. The YAG crystal is doped by allowing atoms of neodymium (Nd) to diffuse into it, making an Nd:YAG laser.

Laser action is achieved in a crystal by exposing it to a powerful light, as shown in Figure 8.5. The photons from the arc lamp pumps electrons orbiting crystal atoms into excited states, from which they are stimulated by previously existing laser light to emit more coherent, monochromatic light. The mirrors at either end of the crystal form a light resonator to build up the intensity of the beam. The partially (approximately 75 percent) reflective mirror on the right in the figure transmits the light to an articulated optical arm or to optical fiber for use in surgery.

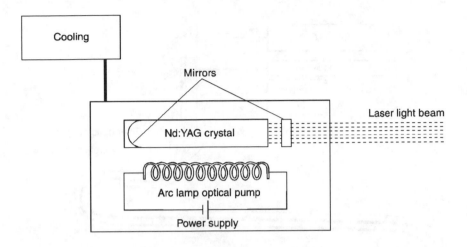

FIGURE 8.5   An Nd:YAG crystal laser

Nd:YAG Laser

Nd:YAG produces light at a wavelength of 1.06 microns, which is just on the edge of the visible band and is considered infrared and invisible. It requires an aiming light, which may be a He-Ne laser that produces red light or a white-light xenon lamp. An Nd:YAG laser apparatus is illustrated in Figure 8.6. Nd:YAG lasers produce power levels up to 100 W and have an efficiency of less than 15 percent, so most of the power supply energy has to be carried away as waste in a cooling system.

Nd:YAG light can be effectively transmitted through quartz optical fibers, a feature that makes them more maneuverable in surgery than lasers that use articulated optical tubes and lenses. Some light is lost by attenuation through the optical fiber, which produces waste heat that is carried away by a cooling gas directed along the fiber, as illustrated in the figure. The quartz fiber is cladded with Teflon and coated with silicon rubber. The tip of the laser can be extended beyond the cladding and cooled with gas to keep the laser light from burning the tip. The gas may also help cool the surface of the tissue to reduce unwanted thermal damage.

The optical fibers have a diameter of 0.2 to 0.8 mm. Because the beam is collimated, it produces spot diameters in this size range. However, the spot diameters are increased somewhat by irregularities in the tip. The bare fiber can be used to deliver energy without the need to contact the tissue. Such an optical fiber is shown in Figure 8.7. However, fiber tips are available that allow one to choose the power density of the light on the tissue. In Figure 8.8, for example,

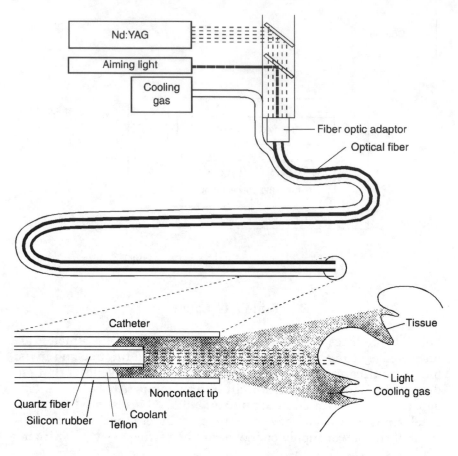

FIGURE 8.6   An Nd:YAG laser

the more blunt tip on the right would create a lower power density than the sharp one on the left. The blunt tip would be used for coagulation, and the sharp one for incisions. The efficiency of a sapphire cutting tip is about 35 percent; therefore, it requires cooling. It is the light emerging from the tip, not the heat of the tip, that cuts or coagulates the tissue.

TYPES OF LASERS

The properties of lasers are determined primarily by their wavelength. The materials and wavelengths used in commercially available lasers are listed in Table 8.1. The laser is also classified by its power level, which will be discussed in the section on laser safety in this chapter.

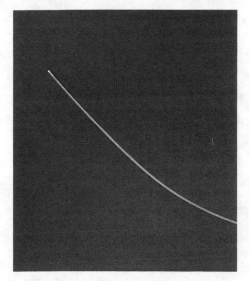

FIGURE 8.7 A noncontact optical fiber used for laser surgery

Laser/Tissue Interactions

The wavelength of the laser determines its nonthermal depth of penetration. *Penetration* is defined as the depth at which the light reduces to 10 percent of its surface intensity. Penetration is caused by the light being reflected off atoms in a process called *scattering*. CO_2 lasers have the least penetration because its light is absorbed by clear water, which makes up a large proportion of tissue. However, argon green light passes through clear liquid and is selectively absorbed by melanin and similar pigments; thus, it achieves a depth of from 0.5 to 2 mm in body tissues. In a clear liquid, such as the vitreous humor of the eye, it penetrates all of the way to the retina. Noncontact Nd:YAG light penetrates the farthest from 2 to 6 mm. This value can be reduced with surface contact probes.

These penetrations locate the point of laser/tissue interactions. On that basis, the CO_2 laser is the most precise because it acts closest to the surface of the tissue in the field of view.

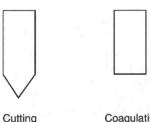

Cutting   Coagulating   **FIGURE 8.8**   Optical fiber tips

TABLE 8.1   Laser Wavelengths and Colors

LASER	COLOR	WAVELENGTH (nm)
Carbon dioxide	Infrared	10,600
Argon	Blue	488
	Green	515
Nd:YAG	Infrared	1,064
Doubled	Green	532
KTP	Green	532
Krypton	Red	647
	Yellow	568
	Green	531
Ruby	Deep red	694
Helium-neon	Red	632
Gold vapor	Red	632
Copper vapor	Yellow	578
Dye laser	(variable with dyes)	
	Red	632
	Green	504
	Yellow	577
Excimers:		
Argon fluoride	Ultraviolet	193
Krypton fluoride	Ultraviolet	248
Xenon chloride	Ultraviolet	308
Xenon chloride	Ultraviolet	351

Source: Absten & Joffe, p. 9.

When tissue absorbs light energy, it converts it into heat, which has the desired effect of vaporizing or coagulating the tissue. However, that heat is also conducted through the tissue and can cause thermal damage. Table 8.2 shows the effect of temperature rise on tissue. The amount of thermal damage depends on the power level and the duration of contact. Therefore, both lateral and subsurface thermal damage can be caused by surgical technique. If the surgeon sets the power level too high, or moves too slowly, undesired thermal damage can occur.

TABLE 8.2   Effect of Temperature Rise on Tissue

TISSUE TEMPERATURE (°C)	TISSUE REACTION
43–50	Observable changes
50–60	Protein denaturing
Above 60	Tissue death
Above 100	Vaporization and tissue ablation
500	Ablation for calcified tissues

To control thermal damage in delicate areas, the laser is applied in short pulses of high peak power. The high energy creates a *photoplasma* that, with very little average power and heat, causes a break in the tissue bonds. *Photochemical* energy from ultraviolet light also breaks molecular bonds in the tissue, leading to tissue ablation with very little heat. *Pulsed lasers* are used in both of these processes.

To protect the tissue behind the treatment area, a backstop of wet sponge, quartz, or titanium may be used.

LASERS IN ENDOSCOPES, MICROSCOPES, AND CATHETERS

Lasers are often indicated when it is necessary to do surgery through endoscopes, microscopes, or catheters. Because laser energy can be transmitted down optical fibers, it can be delivered to sites accessible through almost any vessel in the body, including the alimentary canal, blood vessels, and urinary tract.

Endoscope

An endoscope is used to inspect passages of the ear, nose and throat, esophagus, stomach, upper gastrointestinal tract, and colon. An endoscope is illustrated in Figure 8.9. Afferent optical fibers illuminate

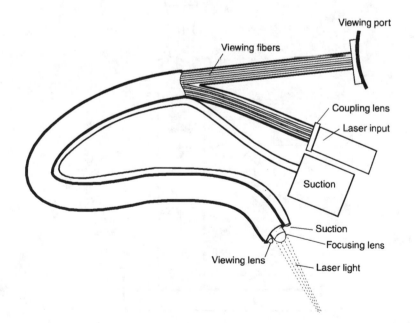

FIGURE 8.9   An endoscope for laser surgery

the surgical field, which can be viewed by the surgeon though efferent optical fibers in the endoscope. The surgical optical fiber is extended beyond the end of the endoscope to prevent heat damage to the endoscope when the laser is fired. To improve the surgeon's visibility, suction is used to aspirate the plume created by the laser treating the tissue. The optical image of the surgical field can be displayed on a television (TV) screen, if the loss in resolution inherent in TV images can be tolerated.

Micromanipulator

In delicate surgical procedures, such as eye surgery, it may be necessary to focus on tissue as small as 0.1 mm in diameter, because the slightest unwanted damage can ruin the operation or have even more dire consequences. In such cases, the surgeon would use a micromanipulator and employ a microscope to guide and focus the laser beam, as illustrated in Figure 8.10.

The laser input is directed to the upper port and passed through lenses that focus it and control the spot size. The aiming light would

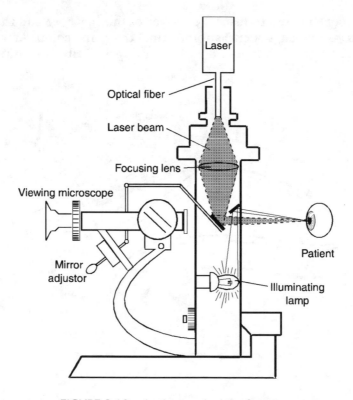

FIGURE 8.10   A micromanipulator for eye surgery

be passed through this port. A standard viewing light is shown at the base of the unit. The surgeon would look through the viewing optics and direct the beam with the mirror manipulator. Appropriate eye protection, which will be discussed in the section on laser safety, is necessary for the surgeon and attendants. An operation microscope suitable for glaucoma and cataract surgery is shown in Figure 8.11.

Catheters

To do laser surgery in arteries and veins, it is necessary to guide the optical fiber through a delivery system, as illustrated in Figure 8.12. The guide wire shown at the center of the cross-sectional illustration is extended beyond the end of the catheter. The wire, which is less than 0.035 inches in diameter, is lubricated so that it can be introduced into tortuous arteries and severely stenosed lesions. The wire guides the larger catheter, which consists of multiple optical fibers for viewing and transmitting laser surgical energy. The injection port may be used to inflate a balloon, as is used in angioplasty. A similar port may be used to aspirate the plume or debris from the surgical field.

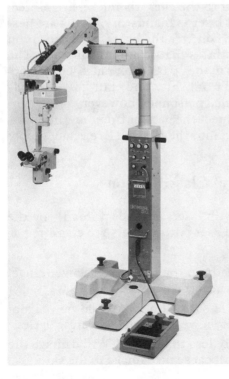

FIGURE 8.11   An operation microscope (Courtesy of Carl Zeiss, Inc.)

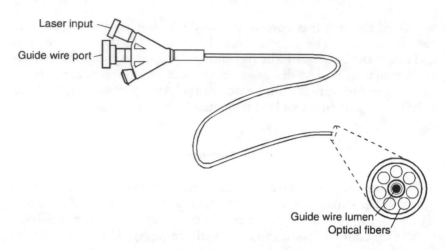

Laser input

Guide wire port

Guide wire lumen
Optical fibers

FIGURE 8.12   Multifiber laser catheter

LASER SAFETY

Laser safety procedures must be followed to prevent unwanted burns to the patient or the staff and to avoid fires caused by the laser beam.

The most serious burns occur to the eyes; therefore, eye protection that is specific to the type of laser is mandatory. Burns are best avoided by a careful operator, who controls the beam and keeps it on target and away from reflective surfaces that would misdirect it. The equipment itself uses high voltages in the 10,000-volt range, but the operator is normally well protected from this. The equipment panels should not be removed by unqualified personnel, however.

The operator also needs to protect the patient from unwanted tissue damage due to heat conduction into the tissue. Here again, proper technique is essential.

Laser Power Level Classifications

The degree of precaution needed with lasers depends primarily on the power level of the light emitted. Laser power levels are classified as follows:

Class I—Fully enclosed, usually in the microwatt power range. No special safety precautions needed.

Class II—Low power, usually less than 1 mW. May be viewed momentarily. Presents a hazard if viewed through collecting optics.

Class III—Power level usually less than 0.5 W. Will damage the eyes if viewed directly, but will cause no damage to the skin.

Class IV—Power level above 0.5 W. Is a hazard to the skin and eyes from both direct and indirect reflection, and can cause fires. Power levels may even be above 100 W.

Eye Protection

Eye covers recommended by the laser manufacturer should be worn by the patient and operating staff during laser surgery. CO_2 laser light is absorbed by clear glass or plastic. Street glasses and viewing optics usually provide adequate protection (check the manufacturer's specifications). Green lenses are usually recommended for Nd:YAG, unless it is a frequency doubled laser. Amber lenses are used to absorb the green or blue light of argon lasers. The wavelength protection and the optical density recommended by the manufacturer should be inscribed on the lenses. The operating staff should have baseline eye examinations to monitor the low-level effects of laser light. Safe, continuous radiation into the eye is set at 0.4 μW. Air Force regulations allow 1.925 mW for up to two seconds. Always follow your particular OR regulations for eye protection when using lasers.

To reduce the possibility of reflected light, shiny surfaces should be blackened. A white enamel surface reflects about 78 percent of the laser light, while a blackened surface reflects only 5.2 percent. Items like metal surgical implements should be covered. Windows should be covered with opaque material to protect passersby. All doors should be closed and a flashing warning light should be activated during the laser procedure.

Fire Protection

Focused laser light can bring any flammable material to the ignition temperature. During surgical procedures, rubbers and plastics can heat up to 4,000° C in one second. Fires can occur in tubing in the patient, especially in an enriched oxygen or nitrous oxide environment. All rubbers or plastics will burn in more than 48 percent oxygen. Therefore, saline water or a halon fire extinguisher should be readily available. (A CO_2 extinguisher would be too cold for human contact.) As with the ESU, flammable anesthetics would not be used during laser surgery.

Alcohol solutions can burn. Facial hair is especially vulnerable in laryngeal procedures because it is close to therapeutic gasses. Oil-based cosmetics should be removed. The hair should be covered with sponges or wet towels. The teeth should be covered as well. During laser microlaryngoscopy, the rubber or polyvinyl chloride tube can be ignited from a misdirected laser beam. As a precaution, it should be wrapped in metal foil or a special laser resistant tube should be used.

A safety standard for such a tube is that, when carrying 100 percent oxygen, it should not ignite after one minute of exposure from a 70 W laser. Caution should also be used when the laser is near any tubing carrying oxygen or a similar gas. The danger is increased when the gas is at high pressure.

Bowel methane gas is also very flammable. Precautions should be observed in the intestinal and perianal area. Gas may be removed by using mild suction, flooding with CO_2, or blocking the anus.

The Plume

A smoke plume that may contain viral or viable particles, vapor, or disagreeable gasses is associated with high-power laser surgery. The energy of the beam not only heats tissue but also breaks it into particles. The plume may be infectious or toxic and, therefore, should be aspirated from the surgical field. It also interferes with the surgeon's visibility. Depending on its size and level of vacuum, the suction tube should be one or two centimeters away from the laser beam. To prevent bacterial and viral infection, an in-line filter on the suction tube or a mask filter of 0.3 μm (ideally 0.1 μm) should be used.

Calibration

The laser should be regularly calibrated for positional accuracy relative to the aiming light. The power level should also be calibrated. Positional accuracy can be checked by noting the location and spot size of the aiming light on a paper target. The location of burns from the laser light should be at the same position. The power level is tested by aiming the laser beam into a calorimeter. This device consists of a heat insulated chamber. The laser beam impacting the calorimeter will raise its temperature in proportion to the power level. The scale on the calorimeter is given as watts of power.

INDICATIONS FOR LASER USE

The advantages of the laser center are its greater precision than any other modality of surgery, the fact that it can be conducted through fiber optics, and its tissue selectivity. The monochromatic beam can be focused to a 0.1-mm diameter and, theoretically, can remove one cell at a time. The color of the beam makes possible tissue selectivity by color, so that diseased cells can sometimes be removed selectively from otherwise healthy tissue. For example, red tissue will absorb red light, heat up and be destroyed, whereas blue tissue will be unaffected by the red light. Fiber optics can be used with argon and Nd:YAG. Where color selectivity and the use of fiberoptics have application, the laser is absolutely indicated over the cold knife and the electrosurgical unit (ESU), although the ESU can be threaded through a catheter as well.

The laser is a thermal knife, however, and can always cause unwanted thermal damage to tissue. The ESU is competitive as a thermal knife. It has the advantages of higher power capability, more efficiency, smaller size, more flexibility, lower cost, and longer established use, especially in general surgery.

It is advantageous to use the laser when catheters are used both in blood vessels and in the endoscopic, laryngoscopic, broncoscopic procedures. The fiber optics are used to deliver light for viewing and illuminating the surgical field, as well as for delivering the treatment energy.

Eye Surgery

In retinal detachment, the color selectivity of the laser is used to pass argon laser light through the vitreous humor of the eye, without absorption, to the retina where it is absorbed. Photocoagulation on the retina results, which stops the tear from progressing into a detachment.

Glaucoma is a disease characterized by an increase in intraocular pressure. Argon laser light may be used to do trabeculatomy on the trabecular (connecting) meshwork. Repeated treatments may be necessary.

In posterior capsulotomy, the Nd:YAG laser may be used to destroy a crystalline capsule, which is located behind the iris and surrounded by a membrane called the capsule. The treatment may be delivered in one to five minutes.

Ear, Nose, and Throat Surgery

The laser has become the instrument of choice for benign lesions of the upper aero-digestive tract. In laser turbinectomy, pressure on the floor of the nose may be relieved and drainage can be improved by removing turbinate or polyps. A sapphire contact probe can be used to deliver Nd:YAG energy to perform the turbinectomy.

In microlaryngoscopy, the laser may be used for precise tissue removal around the larynx through a laryngoscope without significant damage to healthy tissue. Small blood vessels are sealed, decreasing the chance of malignant cell migration. As was discussed in the section on laser safety, a fire hazard exists when an endotracheal tube is used in microlaryngoscopy. Possible complications for the patient due to the placement of the laryngoscope in the airway include tachycardia and hypertensive periods. Patients with heart problems should be monitored very closely.

In bronchoscopy, the use of the laser has introduced new treatments of diseases of the bronchial tree, which is accessible with an endoscope. The CO_2 laser may be used where a rigid bronchoscope would be used, but more flexibility is introduced through the use of an Nd:YAG laser and an optical fiber. Possible complications include hypoxemia, bleeding, and irritation from debris during the operation. The operation should be stopped periodically to check for these complications.

Dermatology and Cutaneous Surgery

Because the CO_2 laser is so precise and because tissue body water prevents deep penetration, it is preferable to use the Nd:YAG laser for many cutaneous applications. The CO_2 laser, however, ablates superficial lesions with great precision and is useful for larger lesions that require higher power. It is competitive with the ESU, which is widely used in cutaneous applications.

The color selectivity of the laser makes it useful in treating pigmented lesions, tumors with dilated blood vessels. Argon laser light is selectively absorbed by hemoglobin; therefore, it is useful to treat hemangioma. However, its limited power may cause the surgeon to choose either the CO_2 laser or the ESU instead.

The color selectively of the argon laser light makes it the instrument of choice for the removal of port wine stains and tattoos. A port wine stain can be lightened as much as 50 to 60 percent with laser treatment. The color is not removed completely, and the lightening may take months after the surgery. Complications include scarring, hypopigmentation, and skin texture changes.

Telangiectasia, birthmarks caused by a dilation of capillaries, can be blanched with the argon laser because of its color selectivity. Healing requires six to eight weeks.

Gastroenterology and Colorectal Procedures

The Nd:YAG laser is preferred over the CO_2 laser for these procedures because it can be conducted through an optical fiber and introduced along winding pathways. Because of its higher power and deep penetration, it is preferred to argon in relevant cases. Argon is used when color selectivity and a more shallow depth of penetration is desired.

The endoscope is introduced into the orifice and manipulated to the diseased area, as guided by depth markings (landmarks) on the endoscope, by optical visualization, or by X-ray imaging. The optical fiber is then inserted into the endoscope and extended beyond the end of the endoscope. This prevents heat damage to the scope when the laser is fired. Suction is required to evacuate the laser plume and enhance visibility.

The major complication of endoscopic surgery is perforation. Perforation at the cervical level would result in difficulty swallowing and moving the neck. Thoracic area perforation would cause dyspnea and shoulder pain, cyanosis, pleural effusion, or fever. Perforation in the lower gastrointestinal tract could cause a burning sensation, distention of the bowel, pain and rectal bleeding, or hemorrhage.

Cardiovascular Surgery

In 1963, P. E. McGuff and D. Bushnell demonstrated that laser energy could vaporize atherosclerotic plaque in arteries. This technique is indicated for obstructions in the iliac, femoral, popliteal, or tibial arteries when the artery is occluded by more than 80 percent.

In this technique, a metal electrode may be attached to an Nd:YAG laser. Depending on the patient's condition, a local or a general anesthetic is used. To insert the optical fiber, a lubricated guide wire, 0.035 in. in diameter, for example, is negotiated about the tortuous arterial pathways under X-ray guidance. This wire is passed through the lesion to be treated. The guide wire provides a track over which the laser fiber can be advanced to the lesion. The possibility of mechanical trauma is reduced by blunting the distal tip of the fiber optic system.

Laser light is used to vaporize the obstruction. Further opening of the vessel may be accomplished by using polyethylene balloon dilation. The balloons range in length from 4 to 10 cm, and they are 4 to 6 mm in diameter. The balloon is placed under the obstruction and inflated for a time interval of 30 to 60 seconds.

If the offending plaque material is not sufficiently removed, two devices are available to prevent restenosis: arterial stints and the Simpson arthrectomy catheter. The stints are metal support tubes that physically prevent the artery from closing. The arthrectomy catheter consists of a cutting element that rotates at 2,000 rpm. It physically shaves the plaque. The position of the cutting element against the vessel wall is controlled by inflating a balloon beneath it. The shavings are stored in a chamber in the catheter and are removed with it.

The introduction of a catheter through the arteries carries the possibility of vessel perforation. Proper lubrication and careful manipulation by qualified, skilled therapists are essential. Careful monitoring is necessary as well.

Neurosurgery

Brain tumors may be treated with the CO_2 laser because of its ability to ablate or excise tissue without damaging adjacent healthy tissue. In the brain, the mere manipulation of tissue is equivalent to causing tissue damage and trauma. With skilled use, the laser is reported to cause less edema and swelling during the healing process.

The laser is also being used to remove tumors from the spinal cord.

General Surgery

The laser is not as widely used by general surgeons as by endoscopists. In many applications, it is competitive with the ESU. However, the fact that the laser is less efficient, less powerful, more costly, more bulky in the operating room and less understood due to a smaller case history data base work to discourage its use in many cases. So much depends upon the skill of the surgeon in the use of any surgical knife, that the selection is often a professional judgement.

ELECTROSURGICAL UNITS

To do surgery, the electrosurgical unit (ESU) delivers, through an electrode, radio frequency (RF) currents in the range of 100 kilohertz to several megahertz. It is capable of making incisions and excisions and performing coagulation, desiccation, and fulguration. It is the most efficient, powerful, and economical of the thermal knives presently available. It is most widely used in general surgery and in cutaneous surgery. It is capable of fast cutting through massive tissue and of effective hemostasis. Its primary adverse side effect is thermal tissue damage.

The original ESU was invented by William Bovie and is illustrated in Figure 8.13. The transformer, connected to the 60-cycle power mains, steps up the voltage, which is then applied across a gas tube. The high voltage during the peak parts of the cycle ionizes the gas, lowering its resistance and thus drawing a current. This, in turn, drops the voltage and extinguishes the gas, which then rises again in resistance. This oscillation occurs at RF frequencies. That oscillation is selected by the series capacitor and primary coil. It is then available for surgery.

When a return plate is used in surgery, the voltage is taken off the primary coil shown in the figure. The Oudin coil is a secondary coil that increases the voltage by transformer action, so that fulguration can be done without the return electrode, as discussed below. For other surgical procedures the patient return plate is used.

During surgery, the RF current exits the relative sharp electrode, dissipating between 50 and 400 W of power into the tissue to make an incision. The cutting electrode is about 0.1 mm thick and contacts several millimeters of the tissue. The voltage, ranging from 1,000 to several thousand volts, sets up a line of small sparks and raises the tissue temperature such that the tissue parts as the cells vaporize.

The electrode–tissue interface is illustrated in Figure 8.14. The cells themselves form capacitors with a conductive electrolyte inside

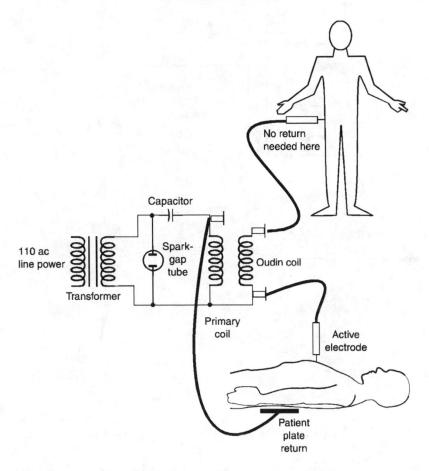

FIGURE 8.13 Spark-gap ESU

separated by a nonconductive membrane from the interstitial fluid. That membrane passes the RF currents into the cell, causing it to vaporize. If the voltage is high enough and is passed quickly enough through the tissue, the thermal damage, as indicated by changes in the color of the tissue, is almost imperceptible. However, if one goes slowly or if the voltage is too low, thermal tissue damage will result. To achieve hemostasis, a certain amount of damage is desirable. The control of this factor is key to good surgical technique using the ESU.

Solid-State ESU

An RF oscillator forms the basis for a modern ESU. A block diagram of a solid-state ESU is shown in Figure 8.15. The device has several modes:

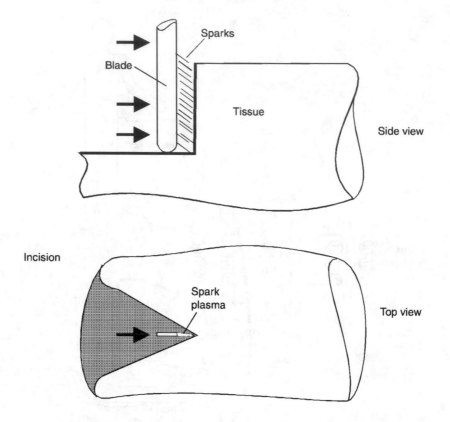

FIGURE 8.14 The tissue–electrode interface during cutting

Cut mode—Pure sine wave, for cutting with the least coagulation.

Coag mode—Pulsed sine wave, low-duty cycle, for coagulating bleeding tissue.

Blend 1 mode—Modulated sine wave, for coagulating as the tissue is cut.

Blend 2 mode—Modulated sine wave, for coagulating as the tissue is cut.

Front panel switches enable the operator to select the mode desired. A solid-state electrosurgical unit is illustrated in Figure 8.16.

Cut Mode

To cut tissue, the switch is usually set to the cut position, as illustrated in Figure 8.15. This connects the RF voltage to the amplifier, which then delivers to the active electrode 1,000 to 8,000 volts peak-

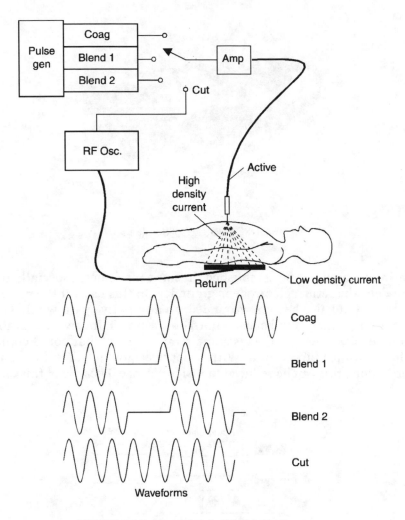

FIGURE 8.15 A solid-state ESU block diagram

to-peak AC at from 100 kHz to about 2 megahertz. High-density currents emerge from the active electrode to do the cutting. A blade electrode, as illustrated in Figure 8.17, is moved through the tissue like a knife to do the cutting. The high-density currents disperse throughout the conductive fluids of the body and return at a low-current density to the patient return electrode, as illustrated in the block diagram in Figure 8.15, to complete the circuit back to the ESU. The return electrode is large in area and gelled to keep the skin resistance low and the region cool (see Figure 8.17). The RF circuit is usually isolated from ground; so if the patient's body comes in contact with ground (through a metal operating table, for example), an alternative path for the return

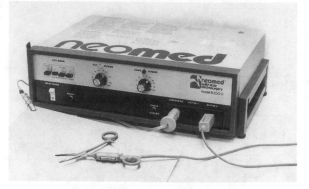

FIGURE 8.16   A solid-state ESU

current would not be established. In some machines, especially older models, the return electrode is grounded. In this case, if the patient's finger would also become grounded, an alternative path would be established, which could cause a burn on the finger. In any case, at these frequencies, there is always some stray capacity that could connect the return lead to ground. With proper design and careful operating procedure, this can be reduced to insignificance. Because of this effect,

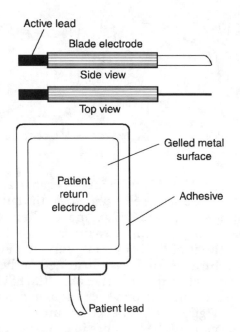

FIGURE 8.17   The blade electrode and return electrode

one sometimes feels a tingle when touching a person who is receiving ESU treatment.

In the cut mode, the ESU continuously delivers its highest average power. Thus, at every instant as the blade is moved along, the tissue receives the same treatment. This results in a smooth cut with no jagged edges.

Coag Mode

In the coag mode, the average power delivered to the tissue is reduced from that delivered in the cut mode. A blunt electrode, such as the one with the spherical tip in Figure 8.18, may be touched to the tissue to produce a coagulum that establishes hemostasis. The power per unit area at the tissue surface is lower than that from the blade in this case. Therefore, the tissue is raised enough to produce coagulum without vaporizing it.

The coag mode may also be established by delivering pulsed energy at a low *duty cycle* (the ratio between the on time and the period between the starting times of successive pulses) of between 15 and 20 percent. Automatically turning the voltage on and off like this slows the cutting process, and allows the heat to propagate into the tissue to form the coagulum. The depth of coagulation depends on how long the electrode contacts the tissue, because tissue damage is caused by heat propagating into the tissue. The edge of the cut will tend to be ragged, and some browning of the tissue will be visible.

There are low resistance paths for the electrical current and the heat, such as along a blood vessel or a nerve going through fat, which can cause deep coagulation. H. Kresse gives the resistivities of the various body tissues as follows:

TISSUE	RESISTIVITY (ohm-cm)
Blood	0.16×10^3
Muscle, kidney, heart	$0.2 \ \times 10^3$
Liver, spleen	$0.3 \ \times 10^3$
Brain	$0.7 \ \times 10^3$
Lung	$1 \ \ \times 10^3$
Fat	$3.3 \ \times 10^3$

These data show that a blood vessel, or blood-filled lesion in the lung, for example, would offer a lower resistance to the ESU currents. This tendency could cause a weakening of the tissue due to the heating, resulting in delayed postoperative bleeding.

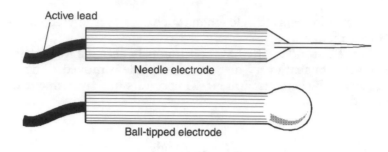

Active lead

Needle electrode

Ball-tipped electrode

FIGURE 8.18   ESU electrodes

Blend Modes

The blend modes are used when one desires to cut and seal bleeders simultaneously. The blade electrode may be used. The lower average power delivered reduces the cutting and increases the propagation of heat into the tissue to coagulate the blood. In this mode, bursts of voltages high enough to establish a cutting spark are delivered at a duty cycle above about 25 percent. In this case, cutting would occur about one fourth of the time; and the rest of the time, the heat generated would propagate into the tissue, creating a layer of coagulum along the incision to control bleeding. The degree of coagulation can be monitored by observing the browning of the tissue. The incision cut may be less smooth than in the cut mode. The sloughing of the tissue under the cut may not be visible from the surface. Less coagulation and faster cutting may be achieved by selecting the blend 2 mode, which may have a duty cycle of about 50 percent. This would increase the time the cutting spark is activated and leave less time for coagulation to occur.

Fulguration

The Latin word *fulgur* means "lightning," and this is exactly what the fulguration spark is. The air between the body and a sharp ESU electrode ionizes when the electric field intensity exceeds 3,000 kV/m. When lightning strikes the earth, the bolt occurs when a charge on a cloud differs sufficiently from that in the earth. With respect to an ESU needle electrode, which is illustrated in Figure 8.18, the body is a charged mass of ionic fluid separated by an insulating layer of skin and air. The inside of the body is the ground, just as the earth is ground for lightning. It is not necessary to have a return electrode to the instrument any more than one would need a return path to the cloud during lightning. The currents travel in and out of the body at the radio frequency of the ESU unit. However, if one does use a return electrode, this adds another path for the current and increases the current in the spark. Likewise, stray capacity affects the size of the spark.

Desiccation

If the ESU needle electrode is introduced into a mass, such as a vascular tumor, the currents will inject power that raises the fluids to above 100° C, vaporizing and dehydrating the lesion. Since lipids and proteins require more than 500° C to decompose, the surgeon has a mechanism to control dehydration. He or she keeps the temperature below 500° C so as to not decompose the tissue while dehydrating it.

Sealing Bleeders

Bleeders up to 2 mm in diameter can be stopped if they are clamped with a metal hemostat. To make instantaneous coagulation, the hemostat is touched with the ESU blade. This process is also done with an *electrocautery hemostat*. This device consists of a conductive forceps that serves as the active electrode. The forceps is clamped over the bleeder, and the current is applied to seal it. The current returns to the ESU through a large-area patient electrode. As illustrated in Figure 8.19, the electrocautery hemostat made by R. Aston in collaboration with Edward Lottick has a sharp edge so that the same pencil can be used to cut tissue and to coagulate bleeders without changing electrodes.

Surgical Technique

The surgeon has control of the cutting and coagulation by the stroke he or she uses. One surgeon may prefer to use a coag blend mode throughout the procedure and control the cutting and coagulation by the force exerted on the blade, the depth of the blade in the tissue, and the duration of contact. The use of the ESU is a refined surgical skill, developed by practice. The different ESUs from different manufacturers produce different waveforms. The waveforms have different amplitudes, pulse duty cycles, and crest factors (the ratio between coag and cut waveform amplitudes). Thus, a surgeon trained on one machine may have to be retrained to use another machine. Some surgeons recommend that, before using the equipment, a few practice strokes be made on meat of the texture to be treated.

The practical consequence of this for attendants is that they should not change the ESU without informing the surgeon. Even different machines from the same manufacturer can differ in subtle ways. Also, calibration of the power levels is done into a test load of fixed resistance. But, in practice, the tissue resistance depends upon its type

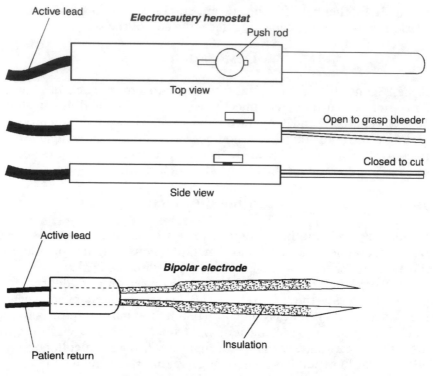

FIGURE 8.19   Two-blade electrodes

as well as the electrode contact area pressure against the tissue. All of these factors influence how much power actually gets into the tissue. The energy then getting into the tissue depends on the duration of contact. In other words, the effect of the RF current on the tissue cannot be controlled completely from the machine; it must be controlled by the surgeon who has experience both in the procedures required and with the specific ESU being used.

Patient Leads

Traditionally, the leads have been classified as either monoterminal or biterminal. This is because some ESUs have only one lead and are used exclusively for fulguration. The lead classifications are as follows:

Monoterminal—An ESU with one wire for patient contact.

Biterminal—An ESU with two wires for patient contact.

Active electrode—The electrode that delivers treatment to the surgical field.

Patient electrode—The large surface area return electrode.

Monopolar electrode—An active electrode that uses a patient electrode to complete the circuit.

Bipolar electrode—Two electrodes in close proximity and of approximately the same size, as illustrated in Figure 8.19, that are arranged so that the current tends to be confined to a small region between the two electrodes. Each electrode is connected to a separate insulated wire but may be packaged in one cable. This type of electrode is used for precise coagulation.

The arrangement of the patient leads on most modern ESUs is illustrated in Figure 8.20(a). The patient leads are usually isolated so that any leakage currents at power line frequencies would be suppressed. The resistance of both leads to ground should exceed several megohms.

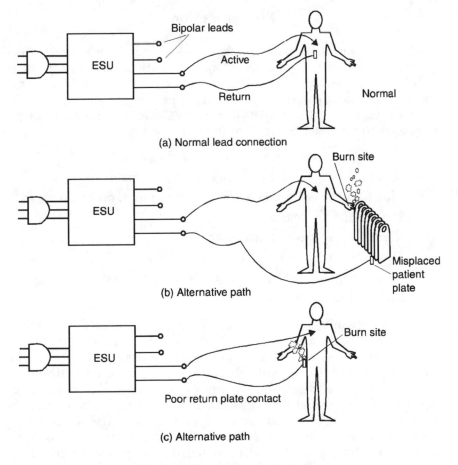

FIGURE 8.20   ESU lead connections

The effect of this would be that any alternative path from the patient to ground would not complete the circuit so as to cause burn injuries at the point of patient-to-ground contact. However, because these are portable patient leads, one might inadvertently ground the return lead and provide an alternative path. For example, someone may set the return plate on a radiator, or it may make contact with a grounded bed or operating table. Safety is most effectively ensured by careful and informed operating procedure.

Some manufacturers provide separate terminals for bipolar leads. These leads often require lower power levels, and the separate terminals provide a measure of safety by making it less likely that the power would be inadvertently set too high.

ELECTROSURGICAL TECHNIQUES

Electrosection

To do both incisions and excisions, a blade electrode or a needle electrode may be used. In both cases, a large-area patient return electrode is required. The essential parameters that need to be controlled in this mode are adequate power, speed of cutting, pressure lightness, and deftness. Cutting levels require 70 W or more. Changes in power level are necessary to compensate for the following:

Differences in thickness and density of tissues.

Differences in the size and shape of the electrode.

Alteration to tissue pH due to inflammation or other effects.

Severe edema or stasis.

Alterations in electrolyte balance.

Tissue changes due to systemic diseases.

Flooding of the operative field with blood or saliva.

Surface dehydration.

Short brushings with a clean electrode is considered most effective. In delicate situations, it may be necessary to wait five to ten seconds between strokes to limit heat damage to tissue. This limits the average power that the tissue absorbs and reduces the likelihood of unwanted tissue damage. Too low a power can cause deep tissue damage because the current flows into the tissue creating heat due to slow movements caused by inadequate cutting. Because tissue damage is proportional to the duration of contact, the cutting electrode should always be moving rapidly while in contact with the tissue. Surgeons say that that it cannot be employed safely with slow, deliberate movements. If the cutting power is adequate, cutting can be done with no co-agulation or thermal damage. However, if the power setting is too low, the deep tissue damage can result in atypical healing of the wound and postoperative pain. As a rule of thumb, if visible sparking occurs, the power is probably too high; and if a noticeable drag occurs, the power may be too low.

Electrosectioning may be done in the cut mode of the ESU, or the blended modes may be used to keep the bleeding minimal.

Electrocoagulation

Electrocoagulation is done by choosing the coag mode of the ESU. The current is applied through a wide-area active electrode and returned through a patient plate electrode. The wide-area contact electrode spreads out the current, making a low current density, so that the tissue is heated rather than cut. In one method, a ball-tipped electrode is put in momentary contact with the tissue and withdrawn. Contact is re-peated as deemed necessary. A scrubbing motion should never be used, according to some surgeons. A light tapping motion is recommended.

Coagulation may also be achieved with a bipolar electrode so the therapist can control the tissue destruction. In this case, the currents are confined to a small region defined by the two electrodes at the tip of the surgical pencil. A large-area return electrode is not needed. This method is effective in confined areas, such as in the brain, where stray currents could cause serious injury to nerves or vessels. Because the currents can be greatly confined, low power levels are effective. Also, the confinement of the currents makes this electrode effective in co-agulating bleeders in fluids such as blood. It is effective in producing hemostasis and sealing off bleeders in soft tissues. It is used to destroy inoperable cancer masses.

Electrocoagulation can cause delayed bleeding if vessels are dam-aged. (Control such bleeding with 30 minutes of direct pressure on wound.) Coagulation is complete when discoloration appears at the treatment site. A popping sound is often heard when the vessel coagu-lates. The current should be stopped as soon as coagulation occurs to prevent excessive thermal damage to the tissue.

Electrodesiccation

Deeply penetrating tissue dehydration can be done with Oudin cur-rents (currents produced by a high-voltage coil that does not require a return electrode). This can be safely used to remove many types of su-perficial lesions in cutaneous surgery.

A dehydrating current is applied to a motionless electrode pene-trating the tissue to be desiccated. This may be used either with or without a large-area patient return electrode, depending on the machine used. Heat radiates from the electrode into the tissue, dehydrating it. It is very difficult for the operator to control the tissue destruction extending beneath the tissue. Only long experience with particular cases can enable the surgeon to predict the effects. This method is particularly dangerous near major vessels, which could hemorrhage from thermal damage, or near important nerves, which could be destroyed by the heat.

The hazards associated with this mode are also illustrated by the case in dentistry: There it is unsuited except in a few clinical uses. It is especially dangerous to the gingival mucosa (gums). It is justified in emergency hemorrhaging in dire cases where local tissue destruction is preferable to severe injury to the patient.

Fulguration

The current is applied by permitting a spark gap by holding the electrode above the tissue. If an Oudin coil is used, a patient return electrode may not be necessary. The spark is moved in a rotary direction. A leather mass, called eschar, is formed, or the tissue becomes charred and carbonized. Appreciable destruction of adjacent and subadjacent tissue need not occur. Fulguration is useful in destroying orifices of fistulae, papillomatous tissue, or fragments of necrotic or cystic tissue wedged between the teeth. It is also useful in controlling bleeding.

TYPICAL USES OF THE ESU

In general surgery, the ESU is used for cutting tissue, stanching , clamp coagulation, and coagulation. It seals gaps in tissues and lymph vessels and protects against toxins, malignant cells, and bacteria. It is a contact surgery, but it is largely sterile. The electrodes can be sterilized before use. Diminution of postoperative pain results because the nerve fibers are not exposed to toxic cell fiber materials.

In urology, a loop electrode is inserted through a catheter (resectoscope) to resect tissue from the bladder, upper urethra, or prostate. A viewing light and rinsing fluid pass through the resectoscope. The surgeon grasps the tissue to be removed with the loop electrode and applies RF power to perform the resection.

In ophthalmology, small coagulating centers can be placed on the sclera of the eye. Diseases such as tumors and glaucoma can be successfully treated with the ESU.

In neurosurgery, bipolar methods are used for sealing vessels at very low ratings, near 5 W. These low powers are adequate for precise coagulation and limit the damage to adjacent tissue.

In dentistry, the principal use of the ESU is for surgery on soft oral tissues. It is also advantageous for treating hypersensitive dentin, bleaching discolored teeth, drying and sterilizing root canals, and doing comparable procedures that involve the treatment of hard oral structures (see Oringer). By electrocoagulation, the ESU can be used for the treatment of inoperable oral cancer.

Contraindications

ESU radiation may interfere with a pacemaker unless shielding, including the coaxial leads, is used. It is contraindicated for (1) biopsy of maxillary antrum and parotid gland, (2) aphthous ulcer, (3) electrolyte imbalance (a high sodium content of intracellular and extracellular fluids causes sparks), and (4) preparation of subgingival trough by electrocoagulation.

Since the introduction of intravenous barbiturates for general anesthesia and the use of nonexplosive anesthetics, the ESU is not contraindicated during anesthesia.

Complications

An uninsulated electrode can cause inadvertent burns to the patient's lips or tongue or to the doctor's fingers. Poor patient electrode placement can cause burns at the contact point due to small-area contact. Alternative paths for the RF current other than through the patient return electrode can burn fingers, for example, if they provided the alternative pathway. This can happen even with the normal ESU illustrated in Figure 8.20(a).

Suppose, for example, that the patient plate is misplaced as shown in Figure 8.20(b). Someone has put it on the same metal surface that is in contact with the patient's hand. A burn, as illustrated, could occur even though the patient plate is isolated and has tested safe. In Figure 8.20(c), poor patient plate contact makes the surface area so small that a skin burn results at that point. Because of the high voltage levels and high frequency, stray capacity can get high enough to provide an alternative pathway for the RF current.

To protect the patient against electrical shock, a three prong plug should be used on the equipment power cord, and the wall receptacle should be checked for proper wiring and safety.

Tissue damage is wider on the corneal layer of the skin than in the papillary body or subcutis, and it is wider still in the fatty tissue. In bone, the thermal layer travels along the periosteum while penetrating slowly under the electrode tip. In severed vessels, the blood recedes and the intima is damaged extensively. The heat flow into the tissue, reflected as its temperature, is approximately proportional to

$1/r^4$, where r is the radial distance from the point of electrode contact. Heating of the tissue causes a coagulated albumin to collect on both sides of the cut. The depth of coagulation depends upon speed of the electrode, the type of tissue, and electrode shape.

RF interference from the ESU occurs because the wires from the pacemaker act like a radio antenna and pick up the ESU radiation. Sensor wires are particularly vulnerable because the RF signal can travel over the wire and either inhibit or trigger the pacemaker inadvertently. If the ESU is being used with a pacemaker, the active electrode should be kept as far away as possible, and the path from the active electrode to the return electrode should not pass through the pacemaker. If the interference has the potential to inhibit the pacemaker, it should be applied for less than five-second intervals to limit the potential downtime. In these cases, the patient's heartbeat should be monitored carefully.

Electrical shock is avoided if the equipment is properly inspected for low-frequency leakage currents. The therapist can avoid shocks by wearing rubber insulating gloves.

The risk of explosion is associated with the use of flammable anesthetics. Explosive colon gas may be neutralized by flooding the colon with CO_2.

Unsterile electrode tips are sometimes used even though this practice is challenged by data. If the skin is not intact, dermatitis can occur from dispersive return electrodes.

A COMPARISON OF THE ESU, COLD KNIFE, AND LASER

The ESU Versus the Cold Knife

When large, rapid excisions in vascular areas are required, the ESU is the method of choice because the advantage of hemostasis more than balances the unwanted tissue damage. When all factors are the same, the knife is preferred because there is no thermal damage and the wounds heal faster.

The ESU Versus the Laser

Considering the CO_2 laser and the ESU, histologic damage is about the same in both modalities if the average power absorbed by the tissue is the same. The cold knife causes less thermal damage than either the laser or ESU. Bloodless excision can be performed with both the ESU and the laser. The ESU is more flexible and less expensive than the laser. Sealing large vessels may be easier with the ESU because of the electrocautery hemostat. The ESU is capable of delivering higher power than the laser and can therefore go faster. However, the laser is more precise because it can be focused down to the size of a single cell.

Thermal tissue damage may be better controlled with the laser because ESU currents can travel down low-resistance vessels and nerves. This could cause tissue sloughing and delayed hemorrhaging. However, skill in use is such a large factor that this would be a weak basis for choosing the laser over the ESU. In both thermal knives, damage depends upon how much energy the tissue must absorb per unit of time. The ESU may tend to make larger hypertrophic scars than the laser, but this factor is also strongly dependent upon technique.

The laser is the method of choice to do color-selective tissue destruction because of the color (or wavelength) of its light beam. This enables it to select diseased cells among normal ones. The ESU cannot make selections on this basis and, in relevant cases, cannot match the selective precision of the laser.

Endoscopic and catheter surgery through fiber optics gives the laser an advantage over the ESU. Capacitive coupling along the length of the ESU catheter can cause burns, especially where it passes through an incision or where the conductor emerges from the catheter and draws an arc. Catheter surgery is done using the ESU. The use of ESU procedures are continued in part because the surgeons have more experience with the ESU—it was used for decades before the laser was invented. The laser is used in gastroenterology, colorectal procedures, gynecology, urology, and cardiovascular procedures.

Safety concerns and the need for strict protocols for use are present for both the laser and the ESU. In both cases, they exceed those needed for the cold knife and require considerable time and expense to administer.

REFERENCES

Absten, G. T., and S. N. Joffe. *Lasers in Medicine: An Introductory Guide*, 2nd ed. London: Chapman and Hall, 1989.

Ascher, P. W. "Absolute Indications for Laser Use in Neurosurgery." *New Frontiers in Laser Medicine and Surgery*. Edited by K. Atsumi. Amsterdam: Excerpta Medica, 1983: 181–87.

Aston, R., and E. A. Lottick. "Electrosurgical Blades for Cutting, Cautery, and Hemostasis." *Proceedings of the 26th Annual Meeting of Association for the Advancement of Medical Instrumentation* (May 1991).

Ball, K. A. *Lasers: The Perioperative Challenge*. St. Louis: The C. V. Mosby Co., 1990.

Carruth, J. A. S., et al. "Clinical Laser Safety." *New Frontiers in Laser Medicine and Surgery*. Edited by K. Atsumi. Amsterdam: Excerpta Medica, 1983: 140–49.

Chin, A., and T. J. Fogarty. "Balloons and Mechanical Devices." *Lasers in Cardiovascular Disease.* 2nd ed. By R. A. White and W. S. Grundfest. Chicago: Year Book Medical Publishers, Inc., 1989: 217–27.

Goldman, L. *The Biomedical Laser: Technology and Clinical Applications.* New York: Springer-Verlag, 1981.

Kaplan, I. "Past, Present and Future of CO_2 Laser Surgery." *New Frontiers in Laser Medicine and Surgery.* Edited by A. Kazuhiko. Amsterdam: Excerpta Medica, 1983: 7.

Kohl, Martin. "Electrosurgery." *Handbook of Electromedicine.* Edited by H. Kresse. New York: John Wiley & Sons, 1985.

Oringer, Maurice J. *Electrosurgery in Dentistry.* Philadelphia: W. B. Saunders Company, 1975.

Pollack, S. V., *Electrosurgery of the Skin.* New York: Churchill Livingston, 1991.

Sebben, Jack E. *Cutaneous Electrosurgery.* Chicago: Year Book Medical Publishers, Inc., 1989.

White, R. A. and W. S. Grundfest. *Lasers in Cardiovascular Disease.* 2nd ed. Chicago: Year Book Medical Publishers, Inc., 1989.

EXERCISES

1. Name the inventor of the ESU, and give the year.
2. Name the inventor of the laser, and give the year.
3. What is the physical process by which the cold knife makes an incision?
4. Name three physical processes by which electronic devices make a surgical incision.
5. Give two terms for removing tissue by cutting it.
6. What is the difference between coagulation and desiccation?
7. Why is the laser potentially the most precise of the cutting instruments?
8. In the lasing process, what causes an electron to rise to an excited state?
9. What is the relationship between the stimulating photons and the laser light emitted from an atom?
10. What does coherent light mean?
11. What does it mean when two light photons are monochromatic?
12. Draw a block diagram of a CO_2 laser for surgery.
13. What is the approximate efficiency of a CO_2 laser?
14. What makes the CO_2 laser relatively akward to manipulate?
15. Why is a helium-neon laser used with the CO_2 laser?

16. To what diameter can a CO_2 laser be focused?

17. Why is the TM_{00} mode used for the laser beam?

18. A focused 50-W laser beam produces a spot size of 0.5 mm in diameter. Calculate the power density in W/m^2 at the spot.

19. How does the surgeon adjust the spot size?

20. What is the purpose of making a large spot size on the tissue being treated by the laser beam?

21. What are the contents of the laser plume?

22. How close should the aspirator be to the plume?

23. What size filter should be used to remove harmful particles from the laser plume?

24. Why are mirrors used at either end of a crystal laser?

25. Why is the surgical tip of a Nd:YAG laser more flexible than the surgical tip on a CO_2 laser?

26. Why do lasers have a fluid cooling system?

27. How is the optical fiber kept cool?

28. How does an optical fiber contact tip used for coagulation differ from one used for incisions?

29. Why does a sapphire contact tip require cooling?

30. Above what power level will laser light damage unprotected eyes?

31. Up to what power level does the Air Force allow momentary unprotected viewing of laser light?

32. Above what power level is laser light a hazard to both the skin and eyes?

33. For what type of laser beam will eyeglasses offer some protection to the eyes?

34. What two parameters must be obtained from the manufacturer's literature on protective lenses to ensure that the eyes are properly protected from laser beams?

35. By how much is the reflected laser light reduced if a white surface is painted black?

36. Name three hazards of laser light.

37. How do you protect against a fire in an endotracheal tube?

38. What body gas is flammable?

39. Why is a CO_2 fire extinguisher not recommended for an operating room?

40. What advantages does the laser beam have over other surgical knives?

41. How does laser color selectivity make the laser the method of choice for retinal surgery?

42. For what eye diseases is laser treatment effective?

43. Why is the CO_2 laser preferred over an Nd:YAG laser for cutaneous applications?

44. Name three cutaneous conditions that indicate the use of laser surgery.

45. Which laser is preferred over CO_2 for endoscopic surgery and why?

46. What feature of argon may indicate its use over an Nd:YAG beam in endoscopy?

47. Describe how a laser optical fiber is used for cardiovascular angioplasty.

48. What color safety glasses are used for the following laser beams?
    CO_2
    Nd:YAG
    Argon

49. Name five surgical procedures that can be performed with an ESU.

50. For what types of surgery is the ESU most often indicated?

51. What range of powers from the ESU are used to make incisions?

52. What causes the incision in an ESU?

53. What type of waveform on the ESU voltage is used when pure cutting is desired?

54. What type of waveform on the ESU is used when coagulation is desired?

55. What range of voltages might you find on an active ESU electrode?

56. What ESU mode is used when you want to cut the tissue and seal bleeders simultanously?

57. Why are the blood vessels and nerves susceptible to deep coagulation?

58. Why is it not necessary to have a return electrode for fulguration?

59. What procedure should the attendant follow when the ESU in the OR has been changed?

60. Define the following ESU electrodes:
    Active
    Patient
    Bipolar

61. Name five different situations that may demand a change in power level during electrosection.

62. How can too low a power setting cause thermal tissue damage in ESU surgery?

63. What is the advantage of using a bipolar electrode in coagulation?

64. An electrocautery hemostat can seal a bleeder of what diameter?

65. Name three advantages of the ESU over the laser.

CHAPTER 9

Intravenous Pumps
and Catheters

You have already learned about catheters that pass electrical currents and devices into the body, such as those used with pacemakers and in laser surgery. In this chapter, catheters that are associated with fluid flow will be discussed. In particular, this means catheters that are used in intravenous (IV) therapy and catheters that are used to measure central venous parameters, such as pressure, temperature, and cardiac output. Another therapeutic catheter is a dilation catheter for doing balloon angioplasty. It is illustrated in Figure 9.1.

Two developments in the 1970s have made this topic considerably more complex: (1) the introduction of central venous catheters and (2) the invention of the microprocessor, which made it possible to make more sophisticated IV pumps and controllers. The physical fundamentals of these pumps and catheters will be presented here.

Previous discussions in this text have dealt mostly with electronic devices and concepts. Now the same type of discussion will be made with fluidic devices and concepts. This is simplified by the fact that a strict analogy holds in that voltage is analogous to pressure and current is analogous to fluid flow. Circulation of blood and its pressure and flow rate are among the most vital parameters in the body. Thus, a review of how the heart develops pressure and maintains the cardiac output of blood is presented first.

PUMPING ACTION OF THE HEART

The heart is composed of myocardial muscle cells and pacemaker cells that are arranged in a network that allows the rapid transmission of electrical impulses. Unlike other cells, the pacemaker cells spontaneously depolarize, causing myocardial muscle contraction. As illus-

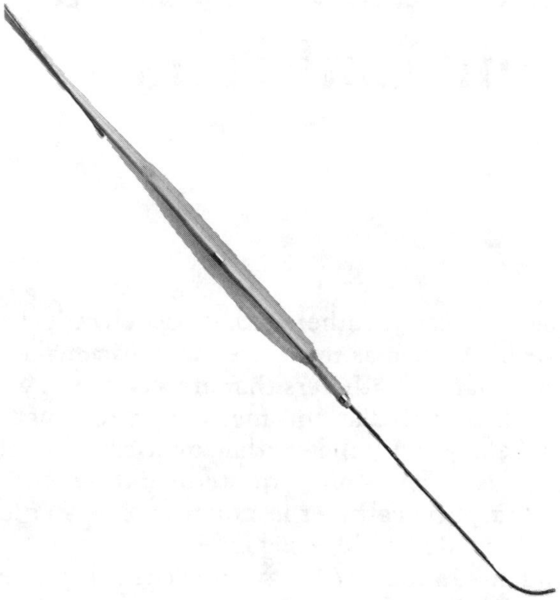

FIGURE 9.1   A dilation catheter (Courtesy of Advanced Cardiovascular Systems)

trated in Figure 9.2, the myocardium consists of four pumping chambers: the right atrium (RA), the left atrium (LA), the right ventricle (RV), and the left ventricle (LV). Blood is circulated through the system by the periodic contraction and relaxation of the cardiac muscle. This electrical and mechanical process is described here.

The electrical depolarization of the heart, a process described in Chapter 3, produces an electrocardiogram (ECG), which is illustrated in the middle of Figure 9.3. Atrial contraction occurs in response to the depolarization wave generated by the sinus node, seen on the ECG as the *P* wave. The atria contract at the end of ventricular relaxation, contributing the last 20 percent of blood (atrial kick) through the tricuspid and mitral valves to the ventricles before they contract. The tricuspid and mitral valves (illustrated in Figure 9.2) are one-way valves that operate such that when the pressure in the atria is greater than the pressure in the ventricles, the valves are forced open like a door.

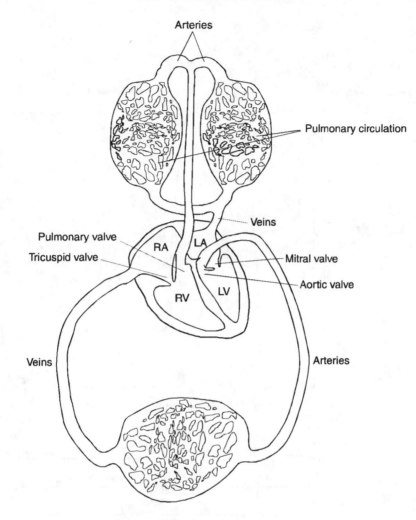

FIGURE 9.2 The circulation system

When the pressure is reversed, such that it is greater in the ventricle than in the atrium, the valve is forced shut, like a door closing against its molding strip. The mitral and tricuspid valves close immediately before systole and the opening of the aortic valve. The mitral valve closes before the aortic valve because pulmonary pressure is less than aortic pressure. The *first heart sound (S₁)* occurs due to vibrations caused by the sudden cessation of blood flow after the closure of the tricuspid and mitral valves.

After all of the blood has been pushed into the ventricles, pressure builds in the ventricles and they gear up to eject. This is the period of isovolumetric contraction. When ventricular pressures become greater

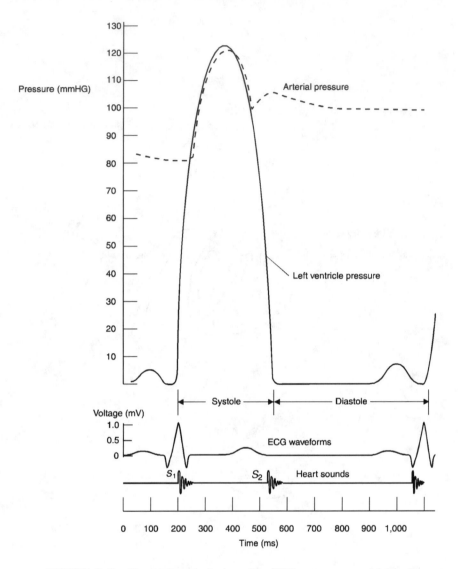

FIGURE 9.3 Correlation between the ECG, pressure, and heart sounds

than the pressure in the pulmonary artery and aorta, the ventricles contract. The RV forces open the one-way pulmonary valve and snaps shut the tricuspid valve. This drives blood into the pulmonary circulation. At the same time, the LV contracts, forcing blood through the aortic valve into the aorta and systemic circulation. After the aortic valve opens (see Figure 9.3), the aortic pressure rises from its diastolic value of approximately 80 mmHg to its systolic value of approximately 120 mmHg. This phase of the cardiac cycle is called *systole*, or the period of ventricular contraction. Ventricular contraction immediately follows the *QRS* complex on the ECG waveform. The *QRS* complex signifies ventricular depolarization.

During the *T* wave, the heart muscle repolarizes, and the RV and LV relax. As ventricular pressure falls below arterial pressures, the aortic valve snaps shut. The sound associated with that event makes the *second heart sound (S₂)*. S_2 occurs due to vibrations caused by the sudden deceleration of blood caused by the closure of the aortic and pulmonary valves. This marks the end of ventricular systole and the beginning of *diastole* (ventricular relaxation). During this period, the one-way tricuspid and mitral valves open, the ventricles fill, and another cardiac cycle begins.

Figure 9.3 shows the LV and arterial pressure waveform as a function of time. The peak value is called the *systolic pressure*, because it occurs during systole. The *diastolic pressure* is the value that occurs at the end of diastole. The dicrotic notch in the arterial pressure wave is caused by reverberations following the snapping shut of the aortic valve.

FLUIDICS OF IV UNITS

Fluid is caused to flow in a blood vessel by the difference in pressure at either end of it. In Figure 9.4, if the pressure P_1 is higher than the pressure P_2, the fluid will flow from left to right. The flow rate, *F*, of the fluid increases in proportion to the pressure difference. The formula is

$$F = \frac{P_1 - P_2}{R} \tag{9.1}$$

where *R* is the fluid resistance. If the resistance doubles, the flow will be cut in half. In other words, the flow is inversely proportional to the resistance. Equation (9.1) proves that the pressure difference in fluids is analogous to the voltage difference in an electrical circuit, and that the flow of fluid is analogous to current. This follows mathematically because the equation has the same mathematical form as Ohm's Law for electrical current, Equation (1.6). Thus, Equation (9.1) is called Ohm's Law for fluids.

The resistance of a vessel, or tube as illustrated in Figure 9.4, increases as the tube becomes longer. Also, a higher viscosity of the fluid causes the resistance to increase. The resistance is most sensitive to the radius of the vessel or tube. In fact, the proportion of the fluid contacting the vessel walls where the resistance is greatest is inversely proportional to the square of the radius. Thus, a larger radius tends to decrease resistance. In addition, the volume of fluid passed by the vessel is proportional to the square of the radius; this effect decreases re-

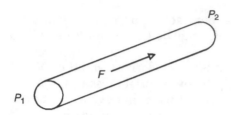

FIGURE 9.4   Pressure and flow

sistance. The two effects act cumulatively to reduce the resistance inversely to the fourth power of the radius, as given by the formula

$$R = 8\eta \frac{L}{\pi r^4}$$

(9.2)

where r is the radius, L the length, and η is the viscosity of the fluid.

This equation is an expression of the fact that the resistance of a catheter or IV needle is dependent on the viscosity of the fluid. For example, an IV needle presents more resistance to blood being passed through it than saline because blood is more viscous. Also, if the length of the needle is doubled, the resistance will double as well; in fact, the resistance is proportional to the length.

Again, if the radius of the needle is reduced by 1/2, the resistance will increase by 16 times, because it is inversely proportional to the fourth power. One implication of this relationship is that if the tubing is pinched, thereby decreasing its diameter (double the radius), the resistance will increase rapidly. Likewise, if a thrombus or a clot of blood adhering to the wall of a needle or catheter forms, it will increase the resistance of the tubing to the fluid flow. In other words, to maintain the same flow rate, the pressure would have to be increased.

During the administration of IV fluids, the solution is elevated in a bottle (or plastic container) above the patient as illustrated in Figure 9.5. In this case, the pressure at the orifice of the tube is caused by the weight of the column of fluid above it. The length of the column is h on the figure. Only the fluid within the dotted line contributes to the weight that presses on the orifice. So it doesn't matter how wide the container is, but only how high the fluid is in the container. The most graphic units for the pressure in an IV tube are centimeters of water (cm of H_2O). However many centimeters high the fluid column is, that equals the pressure in cm of H_2O. Often, this pressure is expressed in pounds per square inch (psi) or in millimeters of mercury (mmHg). The conversion factors are as follows:

1 cm of H_2O = 0.01422 psi (at 4° C)

1 mm of Hg = 0.01934 psi (at 0° C)

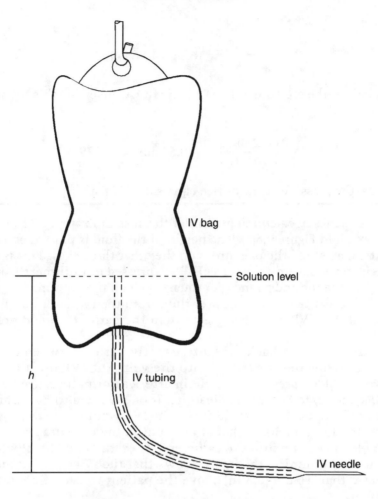

FIGURE 9.5 IV solution container and tubing

The first conversion factor allows the calculation of how high the column of solution must be to create a desired pressure in pounds per square inch. This is because the density (or weight per unit volume) of most biological fluids and IV fluids are approximately the same as the density of water.

EXAMPLE 9.1 The fluid in an IV container is elevated 16 inches above the orifice. Calculate the pressure at the orifice in units of pounds per square inch.

Solution There are 2.54 centimeters in 1 inch, so the elevation in centimeters is

$$\frac{2.54 \text{ cm}}{1 \text{ in}} \ 16 \text{ in} = 40.64 \text{ cm}$$

Therefore, the pressure is 40.64 cm of H_2O. Converting this to psi gives you

$$\frac{0.01422 \text{ lb/sq in}}{1 \text{ cm } H_2O} (40.64 \text{ cm}) = 0.5779 \text{ psi}$$

Thus, the pressure at the orifice equals 0.5779 psi.

A series of calculations similar to those in Example 9.1 produces the graph in Figure 9.6(a). The height of the fluid is plotted on the left vertical axis, and the pressure is on the other three axes. This is called the intravenous unit pressure (IVP), expressed in millimeters of mercury on the top and pounds per square inch on the bottom.

In order to obtain a flow of fluid from the IV container into the patient, the IVP must be greater than the patient's blood pressure (BP).

In the veins back pressure usually varies between 30 to 50 mmHg. Thus to infuse fluid into the vein, the IVP must be larger than the blood pressure (BP). BP in arteries normally range between 120 systolic, to 80 mmHg diastolic. If one wanted to have infusion occur throughout the whole cycle, the IVP would have to be greater than the 120 mmHg, so that at no point in the pressure cycle would the blood back up into the catheter. For example, if the BP on a patient is 12.0 mmHg, the figure shows that the IV container must be greater than 16 cm (6.3 in) above the patient to get a flow into the patient.

The rate of flow into the patient depends upon both the height of the fluid and the IV needle resistance. IV needles usually range in gauge size from 19 (0.0285 inch inside diameter) to 22 (0.0163 inch inside diameter). If the IV needle diameter is much smaller than the tubing diameter, then essentially all of the resistance to flow in the IV set is in the needle. (This is true unless the tubing is pinched or has a kink in it.) For a given needle, the flow rate is determined by how much the IVP exceeds the BP of the patient.

A plot of the flow of saline (viscosity, 0.001 Pa-s) for two common needle sizes is calculated using Equations (9.1) and (9.2) and is shown in Figure 9.6(b). For example, if the IVP is greater than the BP by 13.4 cm of H_2O, the flow of saline into the bloodstream will be 0.04 ml/s through a 22-gauge needle. The larger 19-gauge needle would deliver a flow of 0.35 ml/s, a larger value because it is a larger-radius needle.

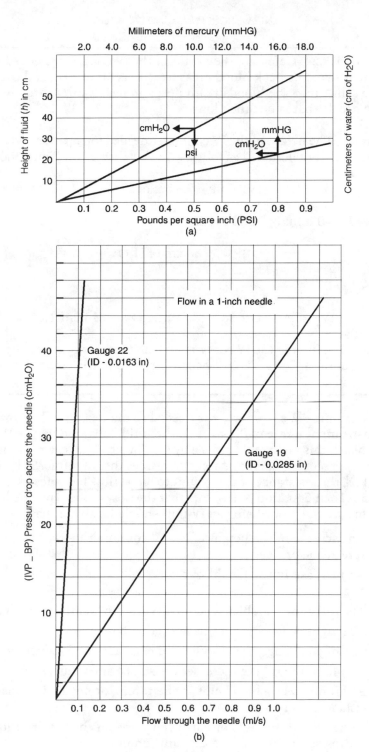

FIGURE 9.6

EXAMPLE 9.2   Calculate the height of the IV container needed when a patient's venous back blood pressure (BP) is 40 mmHg and the flow of the saline into the bloodstream needs to be 0.2 ml/s through a 19-gauge needle that is one inch long.

Solution   The height of the IV container needed for a patient with a BP of 40 mmHg is calculated as follows (in this case, from Figure 9.6(b):

$$IVP - BP = 7.8 \text{ cm of } H_2O$$

Since BP = 40 mmHg, you have that

$$BP = 54.38 \text{ cm of } H_2O$$

and

$$IVP = 54.38 \text{ cmH}_2O + 7.8 \text{ cmH}_2O = 62.18 \text{ cmH}_2O$$

To find the height of the IV container, recall that it is numerically equal to the cm of H_2O, 62.18 cm, because saline is the same density as water.

Example 9.2 shows what is needed to make saline flow into the bloodstream at a rate of 0.2 ml/s. If the fluid delivered by the IV unit were blood, this rate would reduce by one fourth. The reason is that the viscosity of blood is approximately four times that of saline. So by Equation (9.2), the resistance of the IV unit to blood flow becomes four times as great. Then Equation (9.1) shows that the flow reduces by one fourth.

In summary, one using an IV unit should be aware that:

- An increase in the height of the IV container increases the pressure at the orifice.
- An increase in the height of the IV container increases the flow rate.
- The resistance doubles when the IV needle length is doubled.
- The higher gauge needles have smaller bore diameters.
- The higher gauge needles increase resistance and reduce flow.
- A kink in the tubing increases resistance and reduces flow.
- A thrombus or a blood clot in the tubing or needle increases resistance and reduces flow.
- Thrombosed, scarred, or narrowed veins on the patient increase the resistance and reduce the infusion rate.
- Venous back pressure is usually 30 to 50 mmHg.

Often, in order to meet a prescribed infusion rate, the nurse needs to adjust the flow rate to a given value. To do this accurately, a controller is needed.

Controllers

The basics of a controller for monitoring the flow rate of blood are given in Figure 9.7. A roller clamp and a controller unit have been added to the IV unit.

The *roller clamp* consists of a wheel on a rail arranged so that when you roll the wheel in one direction, it will pinch the IV tubing tighter; and when rolled in the opposite direction, it will open a pinched tubing. The roller clamp in effect increases or decreases the line resistance.

The *controller unit* counts the drops of fluid coming from the IV container. If the number of drops falls below a set limit (or, alternatively, exceeds it), an alarm sounds so that the roller clamp can be readjusted to correct the drop count. In an automatic controller, the

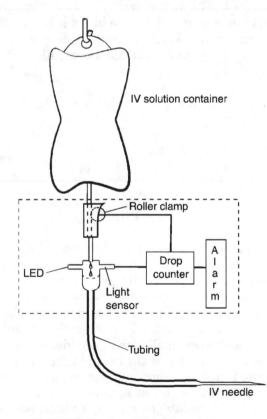

FIGURE 9.7   An electronic controller

adjustment is done electronically. The controller unit consists of a drop sensor, an electronic counter, and an alarm. The *drop sensor* may use a light-emitting diode (LED) that casts a light beam on a light-sensitive transistor. Each drop interrupts the light beam as it passes through. This creates electrical pulses from the light sensor, which are counted in the *electronic counter*. When the number per second falls out of the set limits, an audible *alarm* will sound so that the clamp can be readjusted.

The flow rate depends upon the volume of each drop. Normally, blood drops are larger than saline drops, because the viscosity of blood is about four times that of saline. To find the flow rate in milliliters per minute, it is necessary to know the volume of each drop. This information should be supplied by the manufacturer of the fluid being used. A macrodrip system delivers drops that range from 10 to 20 drops per milliliter. A microdrop system delivers 50 to 60 drops per milliliter. From this information, you can calculate the flow rate from the IV unit, using the drop count in drops per minute (drops/min).

EXAMPLE 9.3   A solution of diluted blood is being infused into a patient. The manufacturer's label says that 15 drops make one milliliter. What is the flow rate if the counter on a controller unit reads 20 drops per minute?

Solution   Divide the number of drops per minute by the number of drops per millimeter as:

$$\frac{20 \text{ drops/min}}{15 \text{ drops/ml}} = \frac{20 \text{ drops}}{\text{min}} \times \frac{\text{ml}}{15 \text{ drops}} = 1.333 \text{ ml/min}$$

IV Pumps

The amount of pressure that can be developed by lifting the IV container above the patient is limited, certainly by the height of the room if not the reach of the nurse. With the introduction of central venous catheters, the line resistance becomes too great to achieve the prescribed infusion rates simply by lifting the bottle above the patient. The resistance becomes high because the catheters are approximately one meter long and have small lumen (inside diameter) sizes. To develop the pressure needed to get the flow required, it is necessary to use either a pressure infusion sleeve or to use an electronic pump.

A *pressure infusion sleeve* is simply a pressure cuff wrapped around the plastic IV solution container. To increase the pressure, one pumps an air bulb and reads the manometer until the proper pressure is achieved. As the fluid becomes depleted, the pressure falls, and it is necessary to pump it back up again. The same idea is used in an *elastomeric pump*, in which the IV solution container is contained in an airtight sac that can be pumped up to apply pressure in the solution.

An *electronic pump* is operated by an electric motor and is capable of providing high pressure for an extended time without readjustment. Two common types of electronic pumps are the syringe pump and the peristaltic pump. A *syringe pump* is shown in Figure 9.8 (see Kwan). It consists of a motor whose speed of rotation can be accurately controlled. The motor drives a screw that presses a piston against the fluid in the syringe. The fluid is then forced through the needle into the blood vessel. The infusion can be very accurately controlled at slow rates, and the volume of fluid is accurately scaled. The syringe is relatively small, usually less than 60 ml, and this factor limits its use in certain cases. Two commercially available syringe infusion pumps are illustrated in Figure 9.9.

The *peristaltic pump* is illustrated in Figure 9.10. It consists of two wheels on the end of a rotating shaft. The wheels come in contact with the flexible IV tubing and push the fluid forward. The flow rate, and therefore the pressure developed, is increased as the wheels are adjusted to push deeper into the tubing and as the speed of rotation is increased. This

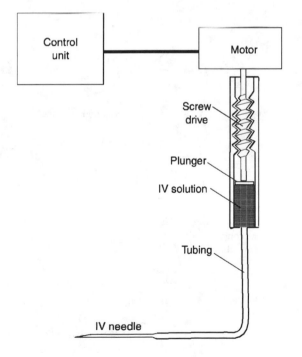

FIGURE 9.8   *A syringe pump*

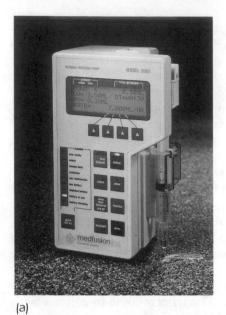
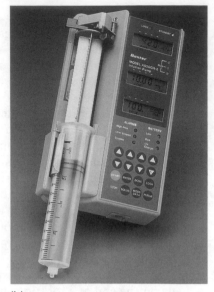

(a)   (b)

FIGURE 9.9   Syringe infusion pumps—(a) is courtesy of Medfusion, Inc.
and (b) is courtesy of Baxter Healthcare Corporation.

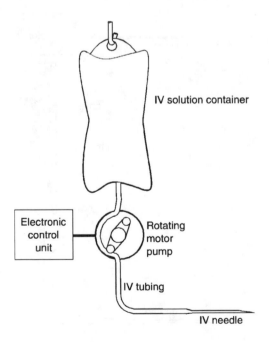

FIGURE 9.10   A peristaltic pump

is called *rotary peristaltic motion,* and its action tends to weaken the tubing after long use. Furthermore, if the fluid is blood, it can damage blood cells (hemolysis). Peristaltic action can also be achieved by fingerlike structures that grip the tubing and are moved in the direction of the fluid flow, pushing the fluid along. This is called *linear peristaltic motion.*

A controller and pump is illustrated in Figure 9.11.

Comparison of IV Devices

An IV unit that consists of a bag elevated above the patient has the advantage of not requiring an expensive, complicated electronic unit, the price of which can range from 1,000 to 5,000 dollars. The elevated bag can be used by a skilled nurse to deliver excellent therapy or nutrition. If higher pressure than can be achieved with gravity is needed, the elastomeric option can be chosen with very little (less than 50 dollars) added cost in equipment. However, it inherently is inaccurate and requires time-consuming tending.

Completely automated controllers that deliver flow rates with an accuracy of 5 to 10 percent will provide rates from 5 to 400 ml/hr (see Beaumont, Kwan). This is the second most economical option, providing that the flow rates are adequate. In these devices, electronically controlled features will sound alarms for open door, low battery, flow rate error, or other malfunction.

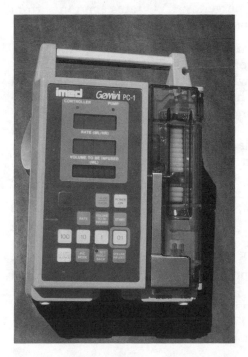

FIGURE 9.11   A unit switchable as either a controller or a pump

Pumps will deliver higher flow rates, from 1 to 1,000 ml/hr. The accuracy is improved to a range from 2 to 5 percent. Commonly available alarm features include warnings for low battery, open door, air in the line, occlusion in the line, malfunction, and whether the settings have been tampered with. These added features come with increased cost, however. To estimate the lifetime cost, a yearly hardware-maintenance cost of 5 percent of the original cost of the unit should be added.

Indications for Intravenous Therapy

IV therapy is used for the administration of fluids or drugs directly into a patient's veins or arteries. Fluid solutions are administered in the following cases:

1. To increase the amount of fluid or to replace or supplement such components as vitamins, amino acids, electrolytes, or lipids.

2. To supply nutrition through dextrose solutions in water. Other solutions include electrolytes, sodium chloride—including saline (0.9 % NaCl), fat, and amino acid solutions.

3. To dispense solutions of blood, including plasma expanders, whole blood, platelet in platelet-rich plasma, and serum albumin.

4. To keep a vein open (KVO) for more convenient administration of drugs or solutions in an emergency. KVO rates can range from 5–10 cc/hr, just enough to prevent clot formation.

IV controllers and pumps may be used to administer drugs when the patient cannot take them orally or when a more rapid effect is desired. IV therapy is indicated when vomiting and diarrhea make oral administration ineffective. IV therapy is used to control the concentration of the drug in the blood and to provide a continuous therapeutic effect.

Infusion pumps for drug delivery have been designed either for continuous infusions, intermittent infusions, or bolus, fixed-mass dosing. Some pumps are designed for patient-controlled analgesia (PCA). With PCA pumps, the patient can self-administer pain medications up to preset dosage and time limits. Special continuous infusion pumps are even being used to inject pain medication into the epidural space. Other pumps are designed for delivery of small volumes of hormonal agents, such as insulin or growth hormone. Syringe pumps may be designed for the precise, intermittent control of drug administration.

When a patient cannot receive nutrition through the alimentary canal, total parenteral nutrient (TPN) is administered by IV, using high-volume pumps that are now capable of rates up to 1,000 ml per hour.

Complications of IV Therapy

The adverse effects of IV therapy include infection, clot formation, fluid overload, escape of fluid from the vessel, and emboli in the bloodstream. The latter two are exacerbated by the use of pumps that can inadvertently apply high pressures.

Infiltration of fluid into the tissue occurs when the needle or catheter is present in the blood vessel and solution extravasates into the tissue. Symptoms include cool skin, edema, discomfort around the site, sluggish IV flow, and usually the absence of blood return. When infiltration is suspected, discontinue the infusion and remove the catheter or needle. Apply ice if the infiltration is detected within 30 minutes of onset and if edema is minimal. Otherwise, elevate the affected extremity and apply warm, wet compresses to promote absorption (see Scherer).

Clots may form in the IV needle or catheter and cause an occlusion. To avoid clots being forced into the bloodstream and causing an embolism by increased pressure from the IV bag or pump, the needle or catheter should be replaced and another vein chosen for IV administration. Another type of embolism that commonly occurs is an air embolism. Causes of air embolisms include air in tubing, loose connections that allow air to enter the tubing, and empty solution containers. In this case, the patient may exhibit a weak, rapid heart rate, decreased blood pressure, cyanosis, and even a loss of consciousness. An emergent nursing intervention would be to place the patient in a left lateral Trendelenburg position, and to notify a physician immediately.

Irritation caused by the needle or catheter on the vessel wall may cause phlebitis (inflammation of the vein) or a thrombosis. The irritation may also be caused by the IV solution or drugs. The affected vein would be warm, sore, and cordlike. Intervene by discontinuing the infusion, removing the needle or catheter, and applying moist, warm compresses. Do not massage the affected area since that may cause further damage to the vein.

Sources of infection include the IV solution, tubing, needle, catheter, hands of the nurse, or skin of the patient. Aseptic technique should be used to prevent infection. To reduce the chance of infection, several precautionary steps should be taken:

1. Choose a site where the needle will remain stable; that is, away from flexion areas, such as at the wrists and elbows.
2. Follow aseptic technique in skin preparation, using alcohol and povidone-iodine or similar antiseptic.
3. Choose a dressing that does not have to be moved excessively.

4. Prevent contamination of the IV tubing by using aseptic technique when changing the tubing, by rubbing injection ports with alcohol swabs before inserting the needle, by properly disposing of used needles and tubing, by changing the tubing at least every 72 hours, and by keeping the needle from contacting contaminants that may also migrate up into the tubing. (To reduce particulate contaminants in the IV fluid, a 0.22 micron end-line filter may be used.)

If an infection of an IV site does occur, assess for symptoms that include swelling and pain at the site. After detecting these symptoms, discontinue the infusion, clean the site, apply antimicrobial ointment, cover the site with a sterile dressing, and culture the needle or catheter. These interventions should be carried out immediately to stop the infection from progressing to sepsis.

Circulatory overload can occur from either an excessive or a too rapid administration of IV fluids. Signs of a fluid overload include increased central venous and arterial blood pressures, venous dilation (especially the neck vein), tachypnea, shortness of breath, and abnormal breathing sounds (rales). Discontinue or slow the infusion to a keep-open rate, monitor the patient's vital signs, and administer oxygen or diuretics if ordered.

Complications associated with the transfusion of blood include allergic reaction, hemolytic reaction (breakdown of red blood cells), febrile (fever) reaction, or disease transmission—including hepatitis and acquired immunodeficiency syndrome (AIDS).

Transfusion reactions require immediate recognition and intervention to prevent further complications from occurring. Upon noticing symptoms such as fever, chills, headache, tachycardia, hypotension, chest pain, dyspnea, wheezing, cyanosis, nausea/vomiting, and circulatory collapse, the transfusion should be discontinued, vital signs monitored frequently, and supportive therapy initiated.

CENTRAL VENOUS CATHETERS

Central venous catheters (CVCs) are indicated for patients who cannot receive IV therapy through a peripheral vein or who need long-term IV therapy, multiple infusions, frequent blood sampling, or total parenteral nutrition (TPN).

The CVC was introduced clinically by Belding Scribner in the late 1960s; this small-bore, single-lumen catheter is called a Broviac catheter. In 1975, Robert O. Hickman modified the catheter with a larger bore. Hickman catheters also come with double lumens (tubes). The lumens of these catheters open directly into the vein into which they are inserted; as a result, blood has a tendency to flow into them. To prevent this, LeRoy Groshong modified the catheter with a closed slit on the tip in 1978. Peripherally inserted central catheters (PICCs), originally introduced in the 1960s, are enjoying popularity again since they can be inserted by nurses certified in the procedure. Triple lumen' catheters were introduced in the 1980s.

The CVC is usually made of a bio-compatible material, such as silicone. The outside diameter is measured in French units, each number representing 1/3 millimeter of diameter. For example, a 3-French catheter has a 1-mm outside diameter (OD), and a 6-French catheter has a 2-mm OD. The formula is

$$OD = \frac{\text{Number French}}{3} \text{ mm} \qquad (9.3)$$

It is important to know the volume of your catheter, especially if you wish to flush it with just the correct amount of fluid. The approximate volume is given by the cross-sectional area times the length as

$$\text{Vol} = 0.087 \text{ (Number French)}^2 \text{(Length in meters)} \qquad (9.4)$$

The volume calculated here is in cubic centimeters (or ml). For example, a 9-French catheter that is 1-meter long would fill with approximately 7.05 ml. (This calculation neglects the wall thickness of the catheter, so the volume given by the manufacturer may be less than this number.)

The catheter may be inserted by the doctor in the operating room or at the bedside if circumstances warrant it. In either case, strict aseptic technique is followed, local anesthesia is administered, and the patient's face is covered with surgical drapes. Those involved in the procedure must wear sterile masks, gowns, and gloves. The patient is instructed not to touch the sterile field. The patient's body and legs are elevated in the bed and his or her head is low (Trendelenburg position) so that venous access is improved.

The CVC is inserted through a subclavian vein or an internal jugular vein, as shown in Figure 9.12. The catheter is introduced into the subclavian vein with the portion tunneled through the subcutaneous fascia of the chest and exiting the skin medial to a nipple. The synthetic polyester fiber cuff is placed about 2 mm from the exit site in order to promote fibrin growth, which helps anchor the catheter in place. The open lumen of the catheter ends in the superior vena cava.

Exterior to the body, the catheter has a lumen hub into which an injection cap is screwed. A clamp is used to prevent the escape of fluids. A dressing of gauze and tape or a transparent, semipermeable dressing is applied to the exit site.

Slightly different than most CVCs, the PICC is inserted peripherally either through the basilic or cephalic vein and is then threaded into

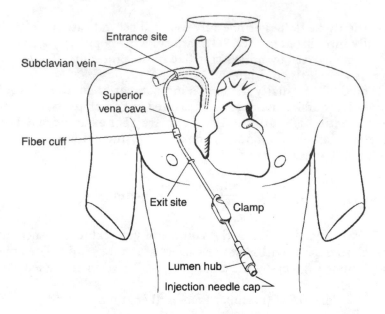

Entrance site

Subclavian vein

Superior vena cava

Fiber cuff

Exit site

Clamp

Lumen hub

Injection needle cap

FIGURE 9.12   A central venous catheter

the superior vena cava using a stylet or guide wire under sterile conditions. The distal end of the PICC exits at the antecubital site. The PICC may be used up to three months for the infusion of fluids, medications, total parenteral nutrition, or blood products. Dressing changes are similar to those for other CVCs.

Because of the back flow caused by the elevated central venous pressure (CVP), blood has a tendency to flow into the catheter and, if allowed to collect, could clot and occlude the catheter. To prevent this, the catheter is filled with an anticoagulant like heparin. This pressure also tends to move any air bubbles up toward the exit site. This tendency can be increased if the patient performs a Valsalva maneuver (closing the nose and mouth and making an exhaling motion), which further increases CVP.

Implanted CVCs

The implanted CVC has a subcutaneously implanted reservoir in a pocket on the anterior chest wall, usually medial to the nipple. The implanted device, shown in Figure 9.13, is known by such commercial names as Mediport, Infus-a-Port, and Port-a-Cath. The port consists of stainless steel, titanium, or other bio-compatible material. A thick rubber self-sealing septum covers a reservoir into which fluids and medications can be injected. For proper infusion, the needle must be passed through the skin and through the septum until it is stopped by the back of the port.

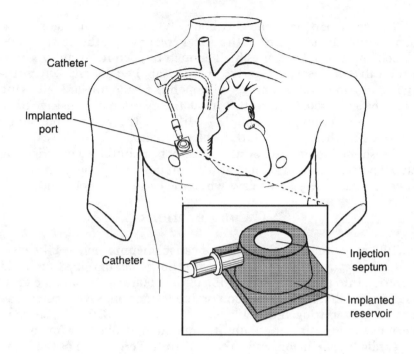

FIGURE 9.13 An implanted CVC. (Clarke & Raffin; used by permission)

The port is used for intermittent or continuous infusions. Only needles designed for the port should be used to ensure the self-sealing integrity. The subcutaneously implanted CVC gives the patient more mobility and is used by home-care patients receiving TPN, chemotherapy, and other medications.

The most recently developed venous access device is the peripheral implantable port, a combination of the PICC and the implantable port. The device has proved to be reliable and safe and have the advantages of less patient maintenance, decreased risk of immediate insertion complications, decreased cost, and lower infection rates. A disadvantage of the device is its smaller size. Patients with an extensive history of prior IV therapy and poor veins may not be good candidates for the peripheral implantable device.

Groshong CVC

The Groshong CVC is distinguished by a pressure sensitive valve at the proximal tip of the catheter. This valve makes it less likely that blood will back flow into the catheter. Therefore, this valve eliminates the need for external clamps and heparin flushes. On the other hand, it increases the flow resistance of the catheter, requiring more pressure to achieve a given flow rate.

The valve portion of the Groshong CVC is shown in Figure 9.14. When no pressure is applied to the distal end of the catheter, the valve is closed unless CVP becomes high enough to open it inward. Assuming the valve is closed, a negative pressure applied distally—by withdrawing a syringe, for example—will open the valve inward, allowing blood to be aspirated. On the other hand, the exertion of a positive pressure—by an IV pump, for example—will force the valve to open outward, infusing the solution into the bloodstream.

Groshong lumen patency may usually be maintained by irrigating with 0.9 percent normal saline (rather than heparin) through the injection cap at least every seven days when the catheter is not in use.

CVC Complications

The CVC may puncture the lung and cause pneumothorax. Likewise, bleeding can cause hemothorax, or hydrothorax can develop from fluid infiltration into the chest. Perforation of the pleura, heart, and the great vessels is possible during insertion or due to motion, severe coughing, or prolonged vomiting. If the lung has been punctured, the patient may experience symptoms of pneumothorax such as dyspnea, cyanosis, tachycardia, hypotension, and a tracheal shift. Perforation of the heart and great vessels would quickly result in pleural effusion, pericardial tamponade, and death.

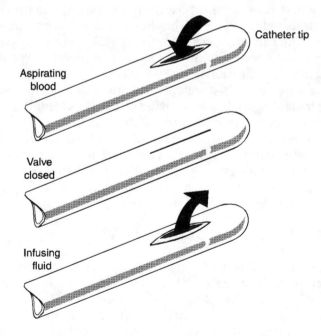

FIGURE 9.14   The Groshong CVC

Symptoms of catheter displacement include the inability to aspirate blood, a swelling of the chest wall during infusion, a leak at the catheter site, and patient pain and discomfort.

Other possible complications include tricuspid valve obstruction or catheter migration. Heart arrhythmias may occur by mechanical or chemical irritation or by electrical stimulus.

With a CVC, the patient is susceptible to microshock hazard because the fluid in the catheter provides an insulated electrical path directly to the vicinity of the heart.

Infection may occur at the exit site or the tunnel along the catheter. The signs of infection are (1) fever and chills, (2) exit site drainage or redness, swelling, pain, or tenderness along the catheter, (3) restlessness and confusion, and (4) hypotension and shock. Staphylococcus epidermis, a common skin organism, is most frequently cultured in CVC related infections. This finding underscores the importance of aseptic technique when caring for CVCs. Treatment of a CVC related infection begins with a trial of antibiotics. If there is no response to the antibiotics, catheter removal may be necessary.

Catheter thrombosis and occlusion may occur when blood in the catheter coagulates or when a fibrin sheath forms around the infusing fluid stream. The fibrin sheath can act as a one-way valve, allowing fluids to infuse but preventing the aspiration of blood. A clot must not be irrigated into the bloodstream, but it must be aspirated or dissolved by a qualified person administering a thrombolytic agent, such as urokinase or streptokinase. Often, the first symptoms of catheter thrombosis are changes in resistance to flow and an inability to withdraw blood from the catheter. Later, the symptoms are those that indicate superior vena cava syndrome and include edema of the neck, face, and arm that are closer to the catheter; nonspecific neck, shoulder, and chest pain; and jugular venous distension.

An air embolism (obstruction of a blood vessel) can occur if there is a break in the system. This break could occur during insertion from a perforation of the catheter, poorly connected IV tubing, or air bubbles infused from air in the solution container. Pulmonary embolism is a thrombus or foreign object (air, placque, fat) that travels via the systemic circulation to the pulmonary circulation, causing complete or partial obstruction of the pulmonary artery or one of its branches. While some patients exhibit no symptoms, others usually present with dyspnea. Dyspnea in combination with apprehension is the most frequent clinical observation in the pulmonary embolism patient. Dyspnea is variable and is related to hypoxemia. Hypoxemia, or a deficient oxygenation of the blood, is not only due to mechanical obstruction of blood flow to an area of lung tissue by the blood clot, but is also related to bronchoconstriction. Chest pain may result from either pulmonary artery distension or ischemia of the right ventricle. Apprehension can result from a reduced flow of blood to the brain. As cerebral hypoxia continues, the patient's level of consciousness will deteriorate. Syncope suggest the presence of a massive pulmonary embolism which causes a transient decrease in cardiac output, leading to hypotension and cerebral hypoperfusion. A pulmonary embolism (PE) may result from the introduction of air into the central venous system. Symptoms of a PE include chest pain, tachycardia, hypotension, dyspnea, restlessness, and anxiety. Complications of a PE may include RV outflow obstruction, low cardiac output, and shock. In addition, air may pass through the pulmonary vasculature and into the LV and lodge in the coronary or cerebral vessels, causing a myocardial or cerebral infarction. An air embolism can cause hemodynamic instability and can be fatal. When an air embolism is suspected, place the patient in the left lateral Trendelenburg position and administer oxygen as needed. Arterial blood gas levels will guide the amount of oxygen needed to keep the partial pressure of oxygen, $^PO_2$ at an acceptable level (>70 mmHg). The patient's oxygen saturation level can also be followed (normal > 95%). The patient should first be placed on the nasal cannula because it delivers low-flow oxygen at concentrations from 22% to 30%. If the patient continues to require more oxygen, various masks can be used to provide oxygen concentrations up to 100%. If the patient continues to exhibit hypoxia, mechanical ventilation may be required.

CARDIAC MONITORING

The heart may be monitored for blood pressure, blood flow rate, and cardiac output in liters per minute. The monitoring may be done noninvasively or invasively in a peripheral blood vessel, a central vein, or the heart itself. The difficulties increase progressively as one moves from noninvasive monitoring to monitoring in the ventricles of the heart or in the lung.

Noninvasive Blood Pressure (NIBP) Measurement

Noninvasive monitoring of the arterial blood pressure is usually done by placing a cuff on the arm as shown in Figure 9.15. The arm cuff is inflated through an air hose that delivers compressed air to it from a compressor. An audio sensor, which is held by the cuff against the skin, transmits turbulent (*Korotkoff*) sounds of the blood flow to the monitor. This arrangement creates an automated sphygmomanometer in which the audio sensors take the place of the stethoscope used to listen for the Korotkoff sounds.

As the timed compressor inflates the cuff, pressure builds, compressing the artery until it closes; blood flow stops, so the Korotkoff sounds disappear. At this time, the instrument records the systolic pres-

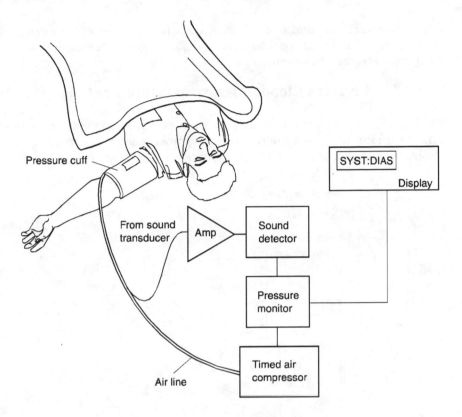

FIGURE 9.15 Noninvasive blood pressure monitoring

sure (SYST). The air is then released from the cuff, and the cuff begins to deflate. The Korotkoff sounds return due to the turbulence as the blood passes through the partially closed artery. When the pressure falls sufficiently that the artery opens completely, the sounds disappear because there are no obstructions to cause the turbulence. The instant they are lost, the instrument records the diastolic pressure (DIAS). Normal SYST:DIAS pressure ratios range from 115:60 to 140:90 mmHG. To ensure accurate readings the size of the cuff should be no wider than two thirds of the upper arm width. A cuff wider than this gives a false low reading, while a narrower cuff gives a false high reading.

The automated pressure monitor has an advantage over the sphygmomanometer because it frees the nurse for other duties, especially when repetitive measurements are required. The monitor may also have an alarm that sounds when the pressure exceeds or falls below either the SYST limit or the DIAS limit, respectively; thus, a critically ill patient can get immediate care. Also, with the automated equipment, the BP can be taken by unskilled persons or the patient at home. The hand-operated sphygmomanometer has the advantage of being less expensive to purchase and to maintain, because it is a simpler device. Also, a skilled user can listen for subtle sound patterns not detected by the automated equipment.

Invasive Blood Pressure Measurement

Blood pressure is measured invasively whenever it is necessary to penetrate the skin to obtain the reading. A typical measurement setup is shown in Figure 9.16. Usually, the pressure at the heart is of most di-

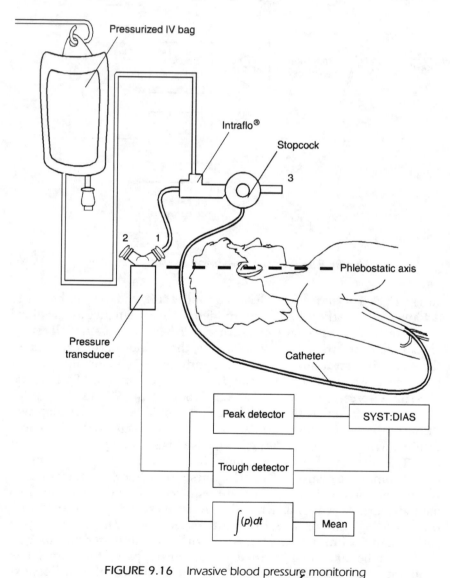

FIGURE 9.16   Invasive blood pressure monitoring

agnostic significance. To get the arterial pressure, a catheter can be inserted into a peripheral artery—either the carotid, femoral, dorsalis pedis, brachial, or radial arteries. However, to get a good reading on the venous side, it is often necessary to thread the catheter through a cephalic or basilic arm vein or through a jugular or femoral vein up to the vena cava or even into the heart itself.

In Figure 9.16, the setup is shown to measure the arterial pressures, including SYST, DIAS, and mean (MEAN) values. The catheter makes a solid fluid path from the artery, through the stopcock and the intraflo device, and into the dome of the pressure transducer. This fluid path transmits the pressure at the artery to the pressure transducer diaphragm, where it is measured. The fluid bag under pressure delivers heparin and saline continuously through the line to prevent thrombus formation and to maintain the column of fluid in the tubing.

To calibrate the transducer to zero, it is placed at the level of the heart, indicated in Figure 9.16 by the dotted line, so that there is no hydrostatic pressure difference. If the transducer were lower than the heart, the transducer would read both the heart pressure and the weight of the fluid in the lines. Thus, the readings would be too high. Likewise, if the transducer were placed above the heart, its readings would be lower than the actual values.

If you want to measure the pressure at a location other than the heart, such as in a cerebral ventricle, the same procedure would be used, except the transducer would be zeroed at the anatomical level to be measured, not at the level of the catheter tip. Remember, the vessel in the body is part of the hydraulic path to point where you want to know the pressure.

To calibrate most types of monitoring equipment to zero, close stopcock 3 (in Figure 9.16) between the patient and the intraflo device; then vent port 2 on the transducer dome to air, and push the zeroing button.

To eliminate air bubbles in the line, first close stopcock 3 and open vent port 2. Then pull the flush tap on the intraflo device to drive the bubbles out of the line. Bubbles in the line between the intraflo device and the patient should be flushed before the catheter is inserted into the blood vessel. The effect of bubbles in the line is to lower the frequency response of the setup so that the pressure waveform will be damped and inaccurate. Damping is the frictional and inertial force that opposes the motion of the fluid in the catheter. The symptom of poor frequency response is a loss of the dicrotic notch on the BP waveform. The same effect can also occur if the fluid lines are too long, or if there is blood in the tubing, kinked tubing, clotting at the catheter tip, or a loose connection.

To prevent air from entering the line, keep all connections tight, including those to the line connectors and the transducer dome. Any dome that is cloudy or leaks should be discarded. Also, the fluid lines should be kept as short as possible.

The electronic monitor measures SYST by doing a peak detection of the BP waveform. Likewise, it measures the pressure at the trough of the waveform for the DYST value. The MEAN is found by mathematically integrating the pressure over one period of the BP waveform. The MEAN is different from the average value (AVG), which is halfway between SYST and DYST. The meaning of the mathematical integral sign in Figure 9.16 is that the MEAN is the average of the averages taken over one period of the waveform.

The accuracy of the DYST and SYST readings should be checked by hand by taking the BP with a mercury sphygmomanometer at various levels. Using two independent techniques to make the same measurement is a good cross-check.

Indications and Complications of Continuous Monitoring

Invasive monitoring of arterial pressure is required in patients who are hemodynamically unstable, such as those with a low cardiac output, when pulses may be difficult to palpate and Korotkoff sounds difficult to hear and in patients who need frequent arterial blood gas monitoring. Invasive monitoring is also required for the evaluation of related therapy.

The major complications of invasive arterial BP monitoring are (1) infection, (2) emboli either from the introduction of air or from thrombi formation, (3) ischemia and necrosis of the extremity used for the arterial line, and (4) exsanguination from a disconnected line. These complications can be prevented through a careful and continuous assessment of the patient undergoing invasive arterial pressure monitoring.

Central Venous Cardiac Monitoring

CVCs are used to measure blood pressure in the vena cava, the RA, the RV, the pulmonary artery, and the LA. This was made possible by the invention of a balloon-driven, multiple lumen catheter by Harold J. Swan and William Ganz in 1970. In addition, cardiac output can be measured in liters per minute by either the thermodilution technique or through the new technique of continuous cardiac output monitoring. Some multiple lumen catheters have bipolar electrodes that can be used to pace the heart. Other lumens carry fiber optic leads that monitor the venous saturated blood oxygen (SvO_2).

A four-lumen catheter for measuring cardiac pressures and cardiac output is illustrated in Figure 9.17. The lead for the pressure transducer articulates to a lumen filled with saline to the measurement port of the

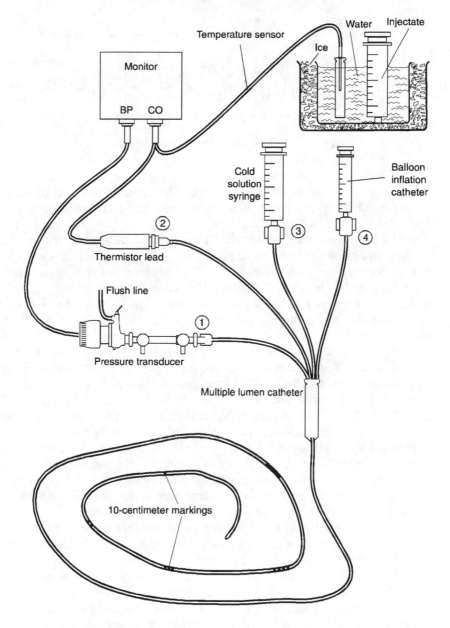

FIGURE 9.17   A four-lumen pulmonary artery CVC (Courtesy of Nikon Koden (America) Inc.)

catheter. The pressure at the tip of the catheter propagates to the external pressure transducer, which is appropriately connected to the monitor. (This is similar to Figure 9.16.) To measure the CVC pressures, the catheter is threaded through the brachial, subclavian, or jugu-

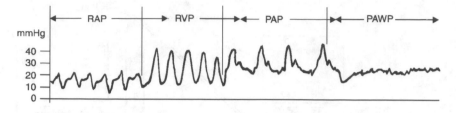

FIGURE 9.18   CVC pressure waveforms

lar vein and into the superior vena cava. The position of the catheter is monitored by observing the pressure waveforms, as illustrated in Figure 9.18.

As the physician threads the catheter into the right atrium, the waveform due to the right atrial pressure (RAP), or central venous pressure (CVP), appears on the monitor. The presence of this distinctive waveform both gives the CVP data desired and confirms the catheter position. Normal RAP (CVP) ranges are from 2 to 6 mmHg. The catheter tip is also radiopaque so it can be tracked with an X-ray fluoroscope.

Further insertion of the catheter through the tricuspid valve and into the RV is accompanied by a change in the pressure waveform on the monitor, shown under RVP in Figure 9.18, which designates the right ventricular pressure. Normal values of RVP are: SYST—20 to 30 mmHg and DIAS—0 to 5 mmHg. At this point, in order to get the tip of the catheter up through the pulmonary valve, the balloon near the tip is inflated by a syringe of air or CO_2 (check your institution's protocol) through lumen 4. The blood flowing through the valve carries the tip with it as it exerts a force on the inflated balloon.

When the tip floats into the pulmonary artery, the characteristic waveform of the pulmonary arterial pressure (PAP) appears, as designated in Figure 9.18. This waveform has a distinctive dicrotic notch. Normal values of PAP are: SYST—20 to 30 mmHg, DIAS—8 to 12 mmHg, and MEAN—10 to 20 mmHg.

If it is also necessary to have an indication of the left atrial pressure, the balloon is left inflated until it becomes lodged in a pulmonary vessel, as shown in Figure 9.19. This causes a hemostasis so that there is no blood flow in the veins beyond to the LA. Therefore, the pressure difference from the balloon to the LA is zero. [This fact is proved by Equation (9.1)]. This pressure measured by the catheter is called the pulmonary artery wedge pressure (PAWP), and it has the distinctive waveform shown under PAWP in Figure 9.18. The normal values of PAWP are from 4 to 12 mmHg.

A pressure, temperature, and ECG monitor is illustrated in Figure 9.20.

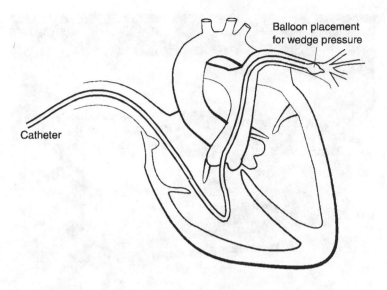

FIGURE 9.19 A balloon-driven catheter

Complications of Central Venous Cardiac Monitoring

Besides the complications associated with CVC insertion as indicated previously, added risks occur because the catheter enters the heart, as well as because of the balloon. The procedure should be done as quickly as possible. The catheter can become soft from body heat and cause convulsion in the veins. Infarction is likely if the balloon bursts. Use of CO_2 rather than air is recommended (Nihon Kodhen). Clotting can occur if the wedge pressure is held over two minutes. Ventricular arrhythmias, such as VT and VF, can occur during the start of insertion until the tip is in the RV. As a precaution, IV lidocaine and a defibrillator should be on hand. The catheter tip can migrate either back into the RV or forward to a wedging position. Both conditions necessitate a repositioning of the catheter. To prevent complications associated with catheter displacement or migration, one must be diligent in monitoring the waveforms to verify the correct placement of a Swan-Ganz[R] catheter. A stat chest X ray should be performed immediately after insertion to verify original placement of the catheter and rule out complications such as pneumothorax or hemothorax.

Inaccuracy in the pressure measurement will result if air bubbles develop in the catheter lumen. They may, for example, dampen the dicrotic notch on a normal pressure wave. The same effect will occur if the tubing to the pressure transducer becomes too long or if the connections loosen. To remedy these problems, the tubing needs to be flushed with a sterile solution, and all connections need to be tight-

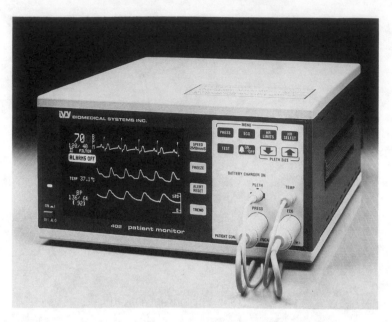

FIGURE 9.20   A patient monitor. (Courtesy of IVY Biomedical Systems, Inc.)

ened. A common source of inaccurate measurements is incorrect leveling of the air-interface port of the system for zero reference. The zero reference port should be at the phlebostatic axis (right atrium). If the patient does not tolerate a supine position for pressure readings, the bed may be elevated up to 20 degrees. Readings should be at end-expiration because intrapleural pressure is static at this time of the respiratory cycle.

A Swan-Ganz[R] catheter is illustrated in Figure 9.21.

Cardiac Output

Cardiac output is the amount of blood ejected by the heart per minute and is the product of the heart rate and stroke volume (the amount of blood ejected with each heartbeat). Cardiac output is monitored with a Swan-Ganz catheter. To obtain a cardiac output measurement, a saline or 5-percent dextrose solution may be either cooled to 0° C or kept at room temperature and injected into lumen 3 of the catheter in Figure 9.17. The fluid enters the right atrium of the heart through the solution injection port shown in Figure 9.22. The bolus of injected fluid cools the blood as it travels toward the thermistor, which is located on the part of the catheter that is placed in the pulmonary artery. If the flow rate is slow, a relatively large volume of the fluid passing the thermistor will have time to be cooled before the injected bolus has passed

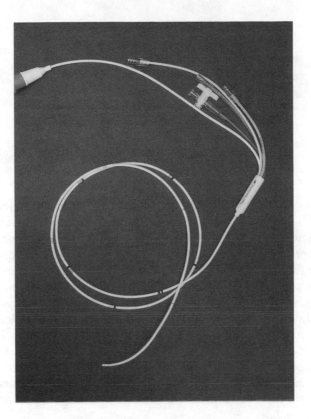

FIGURE 9.21   A Swan-Ganz^R catheter

the thermistor. This is indicated by the temperature versus time curve of the thermistor, illustrated in Figure 9.23. Notice here that a much larger volume of fluid passing the thermistor has been cooled when the blood is traveling at 2 l/min than when it is going faster at 6 l/min. Therefore, the cardiac output (CO) is inversely proportional to the area between the 37° C and the thermodilution curve. This is the shaded area on the 6 l/min curve in Figure 9.23.

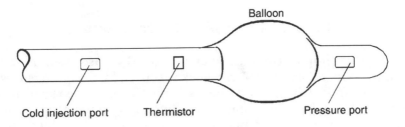

FIGURE 9.22   Catheter ports and balloon

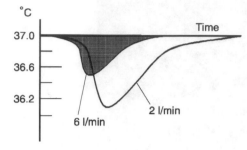

FIGURE 9.23   Thermodilution curve

A cardiac output microprocessor circuit uses the temperature of the injected bolus of fluid and the thermodilution curve to compute the CO value. The procedure for taking a CO reading with the cardiac output computer, illustrated in Figure 9.17, is to cool the injection fluid in ice water for about 15 minutes. This temperature is monitored by a temperature probe connected to the unit. The thermistor connector of the CO computer is attached to lumen hub 2 in Figure 9.17. Assuming that the catheter is properly in place and flushed of all bubbles, the solution is injected into lumen 3, and the CO computer is activated to make the measurement. The normal CO value for an adult is 4 to 8 l/min. If the patient's body surface area (BSA) is known, a cardiac index (CI) is then calculated. The CI is more accurate because it takes into account the patient's size. The normal CI is 2.5 to 4 l/min/m^2 and is calculated as CO ÷ BSA.

When obtaining a cardiac output, the correct injection technique is crucial and determines the accuracy of the cardiac output reading. Therefore, it is just as important to observe the waveform that results from the injection as it is to record the cardiac output amount. A smooth and quick injection of the fluid, timed to begin at end-expiration, decreases variability of measurement. To obtain an accurate cardiac output reading, as with the other Swan-Ganz^R readings, the patient should be in a supine position. If the patient is unable to tolerate a completely supine position, the head of the bed can be raised up to 20 degrees.

Complications of CO Measurement

Besides the complications associated with CVC insertion, infection from the fluid is a hazard. Microshock mediated by the attendant who injects the fluid, which could cause VF, must be prevented by using insulating gloves, by using proper grounding to avoid the conduction of currents down the fluid lumen to the patient's heart, and by draining away the static electricity with skin-to-skin contact.

Continuous Cardiac Output Measurements

A continuous cardiac output (CCO) system (the Vigilance monitor) that utilizes thermodilution has recently been developed by Baxter-Edwards Critical Care Division. CCO alerts the practitioner to changes in cardiac output in response to events and therapies that otherwise may be overlooked. The PA catheter has been modified by the placement of a thermal filament located near the proximal injectate port. This filament is adjacent to the injectate port in the RV. The filament introduces small, repetitive pulses of heat into the blood. These pulses replace the traditional fluid bolus. The changes in blood temperature are read at the distal thermistor located in the PA. Because the monitor is based on the thermodilution principle, it requires no calibration. A CO reading is displayed and updated every 30 seconds, reflecting an average of the prior 3 to 5 minutes of data. The monitor also offers the practitioner the option of the traditional intermittent bolus technique.

Complications of Continuous Cardiac Output Measurement

There are no other known complications associated with CCO other than the complications of intermittent thermodilution CO discussed previously. The small amount of heat released by the filament is well within the safe ranges because the temperature of the catheter never increases above 44 degrees Celsius. Studies show that morphologic changes of the red blood cells begin to occur at a temperature of 48 degrees Celsius after a time of 60 minutes.

SvO_2 Monitoring

The continuous monitoring of mixed venous oxygen saturation (SvO_2) provides the practitioner with current information regarding the adequacy of oxygen delivery with respect to oxygen demand. Bedside, SvO_2 monitoring has been made possible within the last decade by the use of fiber-optic pulmonary artery catheters, which also provide continuous PA pressure, CVP, and intermittent CO measurements. SvO_2 monitoring systems utilize the light of selected wavelengths. The light is transmitted through a fiber-optic filament to the tip of a pulmonary artery catheter. Red blood cells absorb the light and then reflect it back through the other fiber-optic filament to the photodetector. This information is analyzed and the ratio of oxygenated hemoglobin to deoxygenated hemoglobin is determined. An SvO_2 of 60 to 80 percent informs the practitioner that there is adequate tissue perfusion, because SvO_2 is a reflection of the interaction among all the variables of oxygen supply and demand (cardiac output, hemoglobin, SaO_2, and O_2

consumption). An imbalance between oxygen supply and demand would either include a decrease in supply (cardiac output, hemoglobin, or SaO_2) or an increase in O_2 consumption.

Complications of SvO_2 Monitoring

Complications of the fiber-optic SvO_2 pulmonary artery catheter are the same as those associated with the standard Swan-Ganz catheter. In addition, the practitioner must be aware of problems with the fiber-optic system that would cause the SvO_2 readings to be inaccurate. Possible problems include the kinking or breaking of the fiber optics, the wedging of the catheter tip, or a blood clot forming on the tip of the catheter.

Other Capabilities

Some pulmonary artery catheters can even evaluate the functioning of the right ventricle by using the same basic concepts applicable to thermodilution cardiac output determination to monitor RV volumetric measurements. Measurements important in evaluating the functioning of the RV include the right ventricular ejection fraction, stroke volume, end-diastolic volume, and end-systolic volume.

Other pulmonary artery catheters may carry a pacing lead, so that an external pacemaker can be attached, as was described in Chapter 7.

IV THERAPY AT HOME

An increasing number of patients are discharged from a hospital setting to continue with IV therapy at home. Prior to home discharge, these patients have a long-term central line in place. Many patients that were once hospitalized solely to receive IV therapy can now be treated at home. The most common types of home IV therapy include antibiotic therapy, nutritional support known as total parenteral nutrition (TPN), antineoplastic therapy, and pain medication. The condition of home IV therapy patients ranges from bedridden, to ambulatory, to very active. The most important aspect of home IV therapy is patient education.

Patient Education for Home IV Therapy

The teaching process should be initiated while the patient is still in the hospital setting. Teaching should continue and be reinforced in the home setting. The information provided to the patient will be overwhelming at first. Involvement of family members is important for patient support. The most important aspect of home IV therapy the patient must understand is aseptic technique. The concept of asepsis must be understood. *Asepsis* is defined as "freedom from infection." The prevention of infection must be stressed. The sterile supplies utilized in caring for a central line should be reviewed with the patient. The patient should be provided with a supply of sterile gloves, sterile dressing packets, syringes, and other supplies used in caring for and preparing for central line infusions. The patient should be allowed to practice with this equipment in order to obtain competency in aseptic technique. Patient education should include the topics of checking the equipment, cleaning the site, starting infusions, flushing catheters, and changing dressings. The types of complications and their prevention should be included in the patient's education as well. The following lists present a sample of the instructions to be given to the patient.

Home IV Therapy—Checking the Equipment

The patient should be instructed in all equipment used in therapy. The information from the manufacturer's literature and the health-care provider's own knowledge should be used in this education process. All equipment should be checked to prevent complications and assure optimal infusion therapy. The patient should follow these steps in checking the equipment:

1. Make sure that all sterile packages are intact and that sterility has not been violated.
2. Check the glass IV bottle (or plastic IV bag) for any cracks or leaks.
3. Check the expiration date on these containers and supplies to ensure that no date has expired.
4. Check the solution in the containers for any cloudiness, discoloration, or particles present; do not use this solution if present.
5. If an electronic infusion device is to be utilized, review the instruction manual before using. Make sure the infusion settings on the infusion device are correct.
6. If uncertain of usage, phone the physician or home health agency. A peripheral IV catheter insertion is shown in Figure 9.24(a), along with an IV bag for continuous infusion in (b).

Home IV Therapy—Starting Infusions

1. After checking the equipment, remove the IV tubing from the packaging, clamp the tubing and spike the IV solution container. Squeeze the drip chamber until half full.
2. Unclamp the tubing and let the solution flow through tubing (priming), being careful to remove any air bubbles that might be present in the tubing. Clamp the tubing.

3. If an electronic infusion device (IV pump) is being used, be sure it is set at the proper rate. IV pumps are available in various sizes with varying functions. As a patient, you should receive training specific to your IV pump with accompanying literature. IV pumps provide an accurate flow rate and decrease the risk of air emboli. The catheter is less likely to block when using an IV pump because the pump's infusion pressure can be set greater than the maximum venous pressure.

4. Have a syringe with a saline flush solution ready.

5. Using an alcohol swab, wipe the rubber access port on the central line; with the needle-tipped syringe, access the port (cap) and flush it with the saline. If the IV solution administration is to be an intermittent infusion (usually less than 20 minutes), you could place a needle on the end of the IV tubing, swab the central line cap, insert the needle, and then start the infusion as per previous instructions. If the infusion is to last one hour or more, the central line should be clamped, the rubber cap removed, and the end of the IV tubing connected directly to the central line without the use of a needle.

Home IV Therapy—Discontinuing Infusions

1. If the infusion was intermittent (less than 20 minutes), remove the needle with the tubing from the rubber cap.

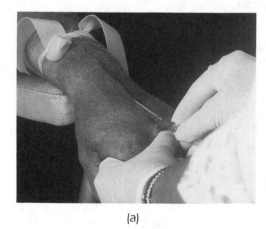

(a)

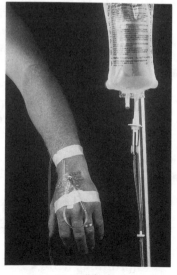

(b)

FIGURE 9.24   Catheter placement

2. Swab the rubber cap with alcohol and, with a needle-tipped syringe, flush the central line with saline. Repeat the process with a heparin flush. The amount of the saline and heparin flush should be ordered by the physician. Common flushing amounts are 2 cc of saline and 100 units per milliliter (U/ml) of heparin.

3. If you had a continuous infusion, clamp the central line, remove the IV tubing, and place a sterile rubber cap on the central lineport. Then release the clamp and flush as in step 2.

Central Line Site Care—Dressings

Site care with dressing changes can be performed with various procedural techniques. The main concern for you the patient is to maintain aseptic technique and follow the dressing change instructions as recommended by your physician. Some standard procedural steps are as follows:

1. When dealing with aseptic technique, always start off by washing your hands.

2. Put on clean latex gloves. Remove the old dressing with care. Discard the old dressing, and put on new sterile gloves.

3. Swab the skin with alcohol, starting at the insertion site and moving outward using a circular pattern. The alcohol swab will help remove dried blood, old ointment, and debris on the skin.

4. Let the alcohol dry completely, then use the same circular motion and clean the site with a povidone-iodine swab.

5. Apply a small amount of povidone-iodine ointment at the insertion site. This provides protection against candida (fungi) infection, which many patients with central lines can develop when they have been treated with broad-spectrum antibiotics.

6. Using aseptic technique, remove the dressing from its packaging and place it over the insertion site. Dressing materials, as with other products in the health-care setting, are constantly changing and evolving with better patient products resulting. Transparent dressings have now become commonplace for central line insertion site care. At times, simple gauze dressings are utilized. The application process is similar in both cases; however, more caution is needed with handling a transparent dressing. The adhesive side of the transparent dressing can easily stick to itself, if its sides touch.

The same methods of site care can be utilized for the implanted port that has been accessed with the special needle and tubing with a rubber cap. The changing and accessing with the needle is the respon-

sibility of the nurse. The dressing changes can be performed by the patient with great care not to dislodge the needle. Sometimes a small (2-
by-2-inch) gauze pad is placed under the access needle to assist with
support. If the implanted port is not accessed with a needle, no dressing
or site care is needed with the exception of watching for anything that
might appear abnormal.

Types of Central Line Complications and Their Prevention

The main complications with Home IV therapy and central venous
catheters are air embolisms, catheter-related infection, and over or
under infusion. The hazard of electrical shock accompanies IV pumps.

It is always a potential danger when the central line has an external access. It is very important to know exactly what type of central
line is inserted; for example, the Groshong catheter is designed to reduce the occurrence of air embolisms. The patient should always take
a deep breath immediately before connecting or disconnecting himself
or herself from the IV solution setup. Prior to connecting or disconnecting, always clamp the central line tubing.

The signs and symptoms of air embolism include dyspnea (shortness of breath), apnea (transient cessation of breathing), hypoxia (low
oxygen content), chest pain, and tachycardia (rapid heart rate).

Catheter-related infection is a serious complication of central lines.
The infection probably occurred from a break in aseptic technique. The
insertion site should be inspected for signs of infection (redness, tenderness, or drainage). Any abnormal signs should be reported to the physician or home health nurse immediately. The patient's temperature will
be checked and, according to protocol, a blood culture test will probably
be done. If the cultures are positive, the physician will start an antibiotic
and the catheter will be removed. The most important thing the patient
can do to prevent infection is to maintain strict aseptic technique.

Infusion therapy was prescribed for a reason. If a patient does not
allow all of the medication or IV therapy to infuse, the patient is interrupting and preventing the appropriate outcome as directed by the
physician. If the central line is infusing the solution very slowly, as
compared to how it previously infused, inform the physician or home
health nurse as directed. If the IV solution has infused too quickly, the
patient should also contact the health-care provider. Under infusion
can lead to poor results of therapy. Over infusion could be life threatening if too much solution has infused in too short a time.

If an IV pump or controller is being used, it is possible to get a
shock from it. To protect against shock, the patient should use either
batteries or a three-prong electrical plug. The equipment must be safety
checked by a support services provider, and the three-prong receptacle

in the patient's home must be checked for proper grounding and correct wiring.

It is the patient's responsibility to inform support services of any concerns or problems. The physicians and home health nurses are there to help. A suggestion in order to assure quality care would be for patients to keep their own patient record. The patient should write down any questions or any problems concerning his or her care. This information should then be shared with the health-care provider.

REFERENCES

Allan, D. "Making Sense of Infusion Pumps." *Nursing Times* vol. 84, no. 35 (August 31 to September 6, 1988): 46–47.

Allocca, J. A. *Medical Instrumentation for the Health Care Professional.* Englewood Cliffs, N.J.: Prentice-Hall, Inc., 1991.

Aston, R. *Principles of Biomedical Instrumentation and Measurement*, Riverside, N.J.: Macmillan Publishing Company, 1990.

Baxter Edwards Critical-Care Division. *Operator's Manual, Explorer Monitor.* Baxter Healthcare Co., 17221 Red Hill Avenue, Irvine, Calif., 92714.

Baxter Edwards Critical-Care Division. *Operator's Manual, Vigilance Monitor.* Baxter Healthcare Co., 17221 Red Hill Avenue, Irvine, Calif., 92714.

Beaumont, E. "Infusion pumps." *Nurse Management* 18, no. 9 (September 1987): 26–32.

Blitt, C. *Monitoring in Anesthesia and Critical Care Medicine.* New York: Churchill Livingston, 1990: 221–25.

Camp, L. D. "Care of the Groshong Catheter." *Oncology Nursing Forum* 15, no. 6 (1988): 745–49.

Camp-Sorrell, D. "Advanced Central Venous Access: Selection, Catheters, Devices, and Nursing Management." *Journal of Intravenous Nursing* 13, no. 6 (1990): 361–69.

Clarke, D. E., and T. A. Raffin. "Infectious Complications of Indwelling Long-term Central Venous Catheters." *Chest* 97, no. 4 (April 1990): 966–72.

Daily, E., and J. Schroeder. *Techniques in Bedside Hemodynamic Monitoring.* St. Louis: C.V. Mosby Co., 1989.

Gardner, P. "Cardiac Output." *Critical Care Nursing Clinics of North America* 1, no. 3 (1989): 577–87.

Gillman, P. "Continuous Measurement of Cardiac Output: A Milestone in Hemodynamic Monitoring." *Focus on Critical Care* 19, no. 2 (1992): 155–58.

Gorny, D. "Arterial Blood Pressure Measurement Technique." *AACN Clinical Issues in Critical Care Nursing* 4, no. 1 (1993): 66–80.

Gullatte, M. "Nursing Management of External Central Venous Catheters." *Advancing Clinical Care* (July/August 1990): 12–17.

Headley, J., and M. Diethorn. "Right Ventricular Volumetric Monitoring." *AACN Clinical Issues in Critical Care Nursing* 4, no. 1 (1993): 120–33.

Intravenous Nursing Standards of Practice. National Intravenous Therapy Association, 2 Brighton St., Belmont, Mass. 02178, 1990.

Klass, K. "Troubleshooting Central Line Complications." *Nursing87* 17, no. 11 (November 1987): 58–61.

Kupeli, I., and P. Satwicz. "Mixed Venous Oximetry." *International Anesthesiology Clinics* 27, no. 3 (1989): 176–83.

Kwan, J. W. "High Technology I.V. Infusion Devices." *American Journal of Hospital Pharmacy* 46, no 2. (February 1989): 320–35.

Lenox, A. C. "IV Therapy, Reducing the Risk of Infection." *Nursing 90* 20, no. 3, (March 1990): 60–61.

Lorenz, B. L. "Are You Using the Right IV Pump?" *RN Magazine* 53, no. 5 (May 1990): 31–37.

Lubenow, T., and A. Ivankovich. "Patient-controlled Analgesia for Postoperative Pain." *Critical Care Nursing Clinics of North America* 3, no. 1 (1991): 35–41.

McKee, J. "Future Dimensions in Vascular Access." *Journal of Intravenous Nursing* 14, no. 6 (1991): 387–93.

Meares, Chris. "P.I.C.C. & M.L.C. Lines." *Nursing 92* 22, no. 10 (October 1992): 52–55.

Noone, J. "Troubleshooting Thermodilution Pulmonary Artery Catheters." *Critical Care Nurse* 8, no. 2 (March/April 1988): 68–75.

Operator's Manual, Bedside Monitor Model BSM-8500A. Number OM.BSM-8500A.ZO5. Nihon Kohden America Inc., 17112 Armstrong Avenue, Irvine, Calif. 92714.

Plumer, Ada Lawrence. *Principles and Practice of Intravenous Therapy.* 4th ed. Philadelphia: J. B. Lippincott Company, 1987.

Reyes-Vargas, V. and P. Gillett. "Pulmonary Artery Catheters Do More Than Ever." *RN Magazine* 54, no. 5 (May 1991): 46–51.

Scherer, J. C. *Introductory Medical-Surgical Nursing.* Philadelphia: J. B. Lippincott Company, 1991.

Schriner, D. "Using Hemodynamic Waveforms to Assess Cardiopulmonary Pathologies." *Critical Care Nursing Clinics of North America* 1, no. 3 (1989): 563–75.

Speer, E. W. "Central Venous Catheterization: Issues Associated With the Use of Single and Multiple-lumen Catheters." *Journal of Intravenous Nursing* 13, no. 1 : 30–38.

Thomason, S. S. "Using a Groshong Central Venous Catheter." *Nursing91* 21, no. 10 (October 1991): 58–60.

Tillman, K. , "Venous Access Devices." *Home Healthcare Nurse* 9, no. 5 : 13–17.

Viall, C. "Your Complete Guide to Central Venous Catheters." *Nursing90* 20, no. 2 : 34–42.

Wickham, R. "Advances in Venous Access Devices and Nursing Management Strategies." *Nursing Clinics of North America* 25, no. 2 (1990): 345–64.

Winters, V., B. Peters, S. Coila, and L. Jones. "A Trial With a New Peripheral Implanted Vascular Access Device." *Oncology Nursing Forum* 17, no. 6 (1990): 891–96.

Woods, S., and S. Osguthorpe. "Cardiac Output Determination." *AACN Clinical Issues in Critical Care Nursing* 4, no. 1 (1993): 81–97.

EXERCISES

1. During diastole, which valves of the heart are open?
2. During systole, which valves of the heart are open?
3. What causes the Korotkoff sounds?
4. When using a sphygmomanometer, how does one know when the systolic pressure appears on the manometer?
5. When using a sphygmomanometer, how does one know when the diastolic pressure is reached?
6. What are the normal ranges of arterial pressure as measured with a sphygmomanometer?

   SYST: DIAS:
7. Name three factors that will increase the fluidic resistance of IV tubing.
8. A plastic IV container of saline is elevated 15 cm above the patient. What is the pressure in psi units that it exerts at the IV needle?
9. An IV bottle of saline is elevated 17 cm above the patient; what is the pressure at the IV needle in mmHg units?
10. What is the minimum height required for an IV bag to infuse a solution into the vein of a patient with a venous pressure of 8 mmHg?
11. What is the minimum height required for an IV bag to infuse a solution into the artery of a patient with a pressure of 120 over 80 mmHg?
12. Will the following factors increase or decrease the flow rate of an IV infusion?

    Higher IV bag
    Longer IV needle
    Higher gauge needle
    Kink in tubing
    Thrombosed needle
    Lower gauge needle

13. How does a roller clamp control the flow in IV tubing?

14. What factors affect the size of a drop of fluid passing through a drop counter in a controller?

15. The manufacturer's label says that 20 drops make one milliliter. What is the volume of each drop?

16. In exercise 15, what is the flow rate of a controller if the counter reads 15 drops per minute?

17. What is the purpose of a pressure infusion sleeve?

18. Name two types of electronic pumps.

19. Name an advantage of using a pump over a controller.

20. What is an advantage of using a controller over a pump for IV infusion

21. What is an advantage of using gravity IV infusion over a machine?

22. What is a disadvantage of using gravity IV infusion?

23. What effect may a peristaltic pump have on blood cells?

24. Name four indications that IV therapy should be administered.

25. Define the following types of IV infusion:
   Continuous
   Intermittent
   Bolus
   Fixed-mass dosing

26. Name four possible adverse effects, or complications, that may accompany IV therapy.

27. If the IV pump occlusion alarm sounds, should you irrigate the IV line contents into the patient?

28. What action should be taken when an IV needle becomes clotted?

29. What is the purpose of the filter in the IV line?

30. Name four steps that will reduce the likelihood of infection, as a complication of IV therapy, through a peripheral blood vessel.

31. What is the maximum time that the same IV tubing should be used with the patient?

32. Name four indications for the use of CVCs in IV therapy.

33. When was the Hickman CVC first introduced?

34. What feature does a Groshong CVC have over a Hickman CVC?

35. In which catheter is patency maintained with heparin, Hickman, or Groshong?

36. What is the OD of a 7.5-French catheter?

37. What is the volume in milliliters of a 6.5-French catheter that is 0.95 m long?

38. What is the purpose of the clamp on a CVC?

39. How does one prevent blood from clotting in a CVC when it is not in use?

40. What is the advantage of having an implanted CVC?

41. Name four noninfectious complications of central venous catheters.

42. Why does the CVC present a microshock hazard to the patient?

43. Name four physiological parameters that can be measured with a multiple lumen catheter, such as a Swan-Ganz^R catheter.

44. Define phlebostatic axis.

45. Why must a pressure transducer be placed at the phlebostatic axis?

46. What factors can limit the frequency response of a pressure-monitoring catheter?

47. Name two adverse effects of bubbles in the catheter.

48. If the dicrotic notch is missing in the BP waveform, what might be wrong?

49. What type of mathematical operation must a monitor do to calculate the MEAN pressure?

50. Draw the block diagram of a monitor that yields the SYST, DYST, and MEAN blood pressure values.

51. Give three indications for invasive arterial BP monitoring.

52. Name three major risks of invasive arterial BP monitoring.

53. Why is a balloon needed on a CVC for monitoring BP?

54. Name two complications associated with a ruptured balloon on a CVC.

55. What precaution is taken to minimize the complications mentioned in exercise 54?

56. Name two methods the physician can use to verify that the catheter is in the RV.

57. What is the maximum time that the catheter should be in place to monitor the PAWP?

58. What happens if the PAWP is monitored for too long a time?

59. Other than with a defibrillator, name a method of reversing a VF.

60. Why does the PAWP measure the left venous pressure?

61. A cold fluid is being injected into one lumen of the catheter, and the thermistor lead of the catheter is being monitored. What physiological parameter is being measured?

62. In which case will the temperature versus time curve be more pronounced—that is, of larger magnitude and duration, for low CO or for high CO?

63. Name one electrical and one biological hazard associated with CO monitoring.

64. What protects the patient from both of these hazards?

65. Besides CO and BP monitoring, name additional uses of multiple lumen catheters.

CHAPTER 10

Ventilators and Pulmonary Function Monitoring

VENTILATION

A ventilator is a device causing air, which may be medicated and oxygen enriched, to flow in and out of the lung at appropriate rates and in adequate volumes. Ventilators are either positive pressure or negative pressure devices. The iron lung, an early form of a *negative pressure* device, creates a pressure less than atmospheric in the lung to draw air into it. The feedback control devices developed during World War II provided the technology that made feasible the *positive pressure* ventilator, such as the one introduced by Motley in 1947. This type of ventilator creates a pressure greater than that in the lung and pushes air into it. Clinically usable devices deliver breaths intermittently and automatically at controlled rates and operate on feedback principles similar to those that control breathing in the body.

Respiration in the body is a complicated process that is controlled by feedback mechanisms in the brain, the vascular system, and the lungs. The physiology of respiration involves three processes: ventilation, diffusion, and perfusion. The term *respiration* is defined in terms of all of these; all of these processes are required for respiration to take place. *Ventilation* is the process by which air is moved in and out of the lungs. The two phases of ventilation are inspiration and expiration. Normally, the external intercostal muscles and the diaphragm contract to expand the lung; this creates a negative pressure to draw air in as the person inspires. Exhalation then occurs when these muscles relax and the elastic properties of lung tissue, along with some muscle relaxation, push the air out. Exhalation is a passive process. The second process of respiration, *diffusion*, occurs at the alveolar capillaries where a gas exchange occurs: oxygen and carbon dioxide move from areas of high concentration to areas of low concentration. The third process of respiration, *perfusion*, involves the process of blood flow and the transport of oxygen and carbon dioxide through the lung and body tissues. Respiration, therefore, is a process that involves the total body. The ventilator only performs one function—the act of moving air in and out of the lungs, or ventilation.

The human body controls ventilation by a feedback mechanism regulated by both nervous and chemical control. Involuntary nervous control occurs in the respiratory center of the brain stem. The three areas in the medulla oblongata and the pons are the apneustic, pneumotaxic, and medullary rhythmicity areas. They work together to regulate inspiration, expiration, and the basic rhythm of ventilation in order to meet cellular metabolic demands. Voluntary control of ventilation occurs only in the cerebral cortex. Chemical control occurs in the central and peripheral chemoreceptors. Central chemoreceptors in the medulla respond to the pH and varying levels of carbon dioxide. Any increase in the partial pressure of carbon dioxide ($^{P}CO_2$) or any decrease in the pH will increase the rate and depth of ventilation to increase the diffusion of CO_2 out through the lungs and out of the body. Peripheral chemoreceptors are located in the aortic arch and the carotid arteries. They respond first to changes in the partial pressure of oxygen ($^{P}O_2$), then to carbon dioxide and pH. Only when $^{P}O_2$ is less than 60 mmHg will these receptors convey the message to increase ventilatory effort. The major stimulus, therefore, for ventilation in persons with normal lungs is $^{P}CO_2$. The major stimulus for persons with lung disease is $^{P}O_2$. There are also proprioceptors in muscles and joints that respond to movements and exercise to increase ventilatory rate. Therefore, range-of-motion exercises increase ventilatory rate, which decreases $^{P}CO_2$.

The process of ventilation requires assessment of several parameters in order to determine adequacy and the potential need for machine-assisted ventilation. Inspiration occurs when the dome-shaped diaphragm in the body flattens during contraction. The external intercostal muscles attached to the anterior ribs also contract to pull the ribs up and out. Air then flows from the higher atmospheric pressure into the expanded lungs with its lower intrathoracic pressure. Inspiration should be a seemingly effortless process. Any use of inspiratory accessory muscles in the neck or upper chest is abnormal and an indication of respiratory distress. Expiration, a passive process, is dependent upon the elasticity of lung tissue and the surface tension in the fluid lining the alveoli. Surfactant helps control the amount of surface tension in the alveoli so that they do not collapse completely. If the surface tension and elastic recoil are inadequate, the accessory muscles of expiration assist in the effort. The contraction of the abdominal muscles to relax the diaphragm and the internal intercostals to push the ribs down will cause an assisted expiration. This is also another sign of respiratory distress.

Definition of Terms

Compliance, the change in volume per unit pressure, is a measure of the ability of the lungs to stretch in order to accommodate increases in air volume. It is a measure of the distensibility of the lungs and thorax. It is not synonymous with elasticity, however. Conditions that decrease compliance include adult respiratory distress syndrome (ARDS), pneumonia, pulmonary edema, pneumothorax, and obesity. Emphysema is a condition that increases compliance.

The rate of airflow from one point to another is proportional to the pressure difference between those points. The *resistance* is defined as that proportionality factor. It is what slows the air down. Resistance to airflow occurs whenever a condition causes an increased work of breathing. When accessory muscles are used for ventilation, resistance has increased. Conditions that increase resistance and, therefore, the work of breathing include copious secretions, bronchospasm, airway suctioning resulting in bronchospasm, chest wall trauma and contusions, a rapid, shallow respiratory pattern, and a small-sized endotracheal tube.

The volumes and capacities used to measure the adequacy of ventilation are illustrated in Figure 10.1. These pulmonary function variables, along with typical values, are defined as follows:

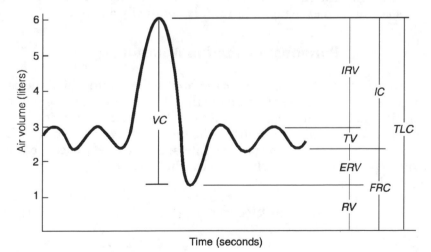

FIGURE 10.1   Pulmonary function parameters

Volumes:

TV—Tidal volume. Measures the amount of air moving in and out of the lungs with each breath. Nominally, 0.6 liters of air are exchanged in involuntary breathing.

ERV—Expiratory reserve volume. Measures the amount of air that can be forced out of the lungs after a normal expiration. This is nominally 1.2 liters.

IRV—Inspiratory reserve volume. The amount of air that can be taken in above the tidal volume. This is nominally 3 liters.

RV—Residual volume. The air in the lung left after a full expiratory effort. It provides for continuous gas exchange even after a forced expiration. This is nominally 1 liter.

Capacities:

IC—Inspiratory capacity. The tidal volume plus inspiratory reserve volume. It is the maximum amount of air that can be inhaled after a normal expiration. It is nominally 3.6 liters.

FRC—Functional residual capacity. The total volume of air left in the lung after a normal exhalation. It provides for gas exchange between normal breaths and keeps the alveoli expanded. It is nominally 2.2 liters.

VC—Vital capacity. The inspiratory reserve volume plus the tidal volume plus the expiratory reserve volume. It is the total amount of exchangeable air in the lung. It is nominally 5 liters.

TLC—Total lung capacity. It is the sum of all of the volumes. It is the maximum volume of air the lung can hold, including dead space air and exchangeable air. It is nominally 6 liters.

Pulmonary Function Monitoring

A spirometer, which consists of a calibrated bellows into which the patient breathes, can be used to measure the *TV*, *IRV*, *ERV*, and *VC*. However, the *TLC* capacity cannot be measured so directly, because of the residual volume of air remaining in the lung. A body plethysmograph, which is a chamber that the patient enters, can be used to deduce this quantity (see Aston, p. 389). If you know the *TLC*, the *RV* and *FRC* can be calculated as:

$$RV = TLC - VC \qquad (10.1)$$

and

$$FRC = RV + ERV \qquad (10.2)$$

These formulas can be easily deduced from Figure 10.1

Neither of these parameters can be used to assess the air resistance. The airway resistance in normal persons is quite low; however, in diseases such as asthma, in which there is severe bronchoconstriction, increased airway resistance occurs. The work of breathing is increased. Parameters that help quantify this are:

FVC_1—One-second fractional volume capacity. The volume of air a subject can exhale in one second using maximum effort. The normal subject will exhale 80 percent of the VC in one second.

FVC_2—Two-second fractional volume capacity. The volume of air a subject can exhale in two seconds using maximum effort.

FEF_{25-75}—Forced expiratory flow. The flow (1/min) taken at levels between 25 and 75 percent of the volume expired.

$\overset{\circ}{V}_E$—The minute ventilation. The volume of air expired (or inhaled) in one minute. This is calculated by the formula

$$\overset{\circ}{V}_E = bpm \times TV \qquad (10.3)$$

where bpm is the breaths per minute.

Pneumatic Ventilator

The simplest conceptual block diagram of a ventilator that has gas-driven (pneumatic) parts is shown in Figure 10.2. The timed compressor

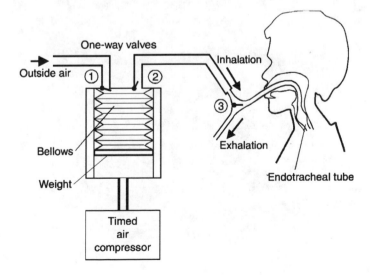

FIGURE 10.2   A pneumatic ventilator

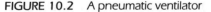

releases air periodically at a prescribed breathing rate. This is a positive pressure ventilator because the device produces a pressure higher than the pressure in the lung in order to push air into it. The device is called a *volume-controlled* ventilator because the volume of a single breath delivered to the patient cannot exceed the volume of the bellows.

Beginning with the patient inhalation phase of the breathing cycle, the compressor feeds air into the chamber beneath the bellows. This pushes the bellows up, forcing the one-way valve 1 closed and the valve 2 open, so that the air is pushed through the spring-loaded valve 3 and into the lung.

During the patient expiration phase, the timed compressor turns off. The metal weight in the bellows falls due to gravity. The suction that this creates pulls valve 1 open and shuts valve 2. Valve 3 also snaps back up, allowing the air expired by the patient to exhaust into the outside air, primarily by the elastic contraction of the lung and the muscles used for breathing. The compressor is timed so that this process continues indefinitely at the desired number of breaths per minute (bpm). A volume ventilator is illustrated in Figure 10.3.

Ventilator Tubing and Ancillary Devices

The patient tubing and ancillary devices are illustrated outside of the ventilator unit in Figure 10.4. Closest to the machine is a *bacterial filter*, which removes bacteria and particulate matter from the air deliv-

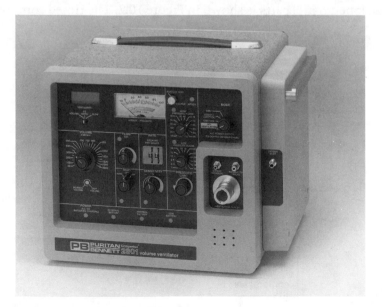

FIGURE 10.3   A volume ventilator (Courtesy of Puritan Bennett)

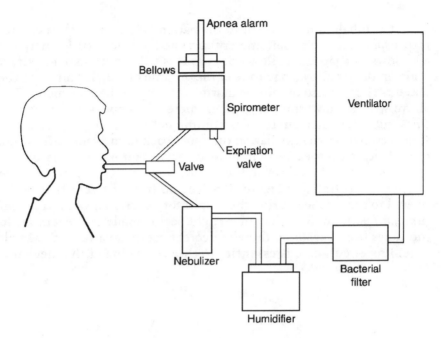

FIGURE 10.4 Patient tubing and ancillary devices

ered to the patient. This will reduce the effect of contamination in the machine and incidents of nosocomial infection. This is especially important because intubation of the respiratory tract bypasses the natural protective mechanisms against respiratory infection.

Next in line is the *humidifier*, which should heat the air up to body temperature (37° C) and raise the humidity up to as high as 100 percent. To do this, the humidifier may inject steam into the airstream. In the humidifier, if the air temperature is not as high as body temperature, it is impossible to achieve 100 percent humidity in the inspired air. This is because as its temperature is raised by the body, the humidity drops. A second mechanism for humidifying air is to bubble it through water in a bottle.

Next is a *nebulizer*, which disperses liquid medication into the air in order to liquify secretions and promote their removal. In addition, a nebulizer promotes lung expansion and relieves bronchospasm. This is done by an aerosol that sprays droplets of medication into the airstream, in the same manner as a perfume aerosol. In this case, the air pressure to make the mist is supplied by the ventilator. A second method for creating the mist of medication is to immerse an ultrasonic vibrator into the fluid medication. An ultrasonic vibrator consists of a crystal that vibrates at a frequency higher than the audible range. It causes small particles of the fluid to eject into the airstream.

The inhalation air goes into the patient's lung, who then expires into a *spirometer*. The spirometer illustrated in Figure 10.4 consists of a bellows in a jar; the bellows rises as it is filled with exhaled air. A scale on the jar allows one to read the volume of exhaled air from the patient. There is also usually an alarm at the top of the spirometer. The alarm will ring a warning if the spirometer does not rise sufficiently. This indicates inadequate tidal volume delivered to the patient. In some ventilators, the exhalation tube goes back to the ventilator where the exhaled air is measured; in these cases, no spirometer is used.

Oral intubation through the oropharynx, the larynx, and into the trachea is illustrated in Figure 10.5. The air from the ventilator is delivered to the trachea during the inspiratory cycle. The *endotracheal tube cuff* is inflated so that an airtight seal is made to prevent air in the lungs from escaping, thereby decreasing the available tidal volume. Proper cuff care is essential to the well-being of the mechani-

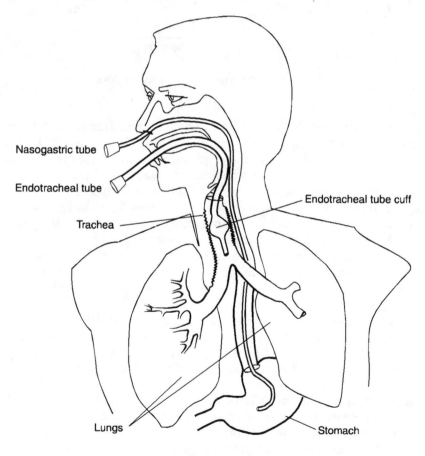

FIGURE 10.5   Oral intubation

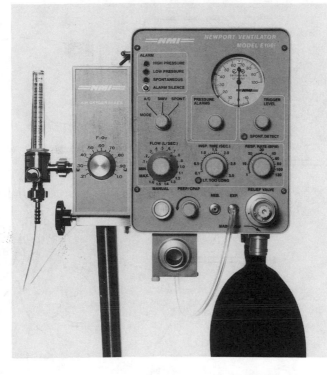

FIGURE 10.6   A ventilator (Courtesy of Newport Medical Instruments, Inc.)

cally ventilated patient. The objective of the cuff is to prevent a loss of tidal volume but with minimal damage to the trachcal wall.

Tracheal intubation may also be achieved by a *tracheostomy*, an operation of incising the skin over the trachea and penetrating the trachea to insert the endotracheal cuff and airway to the lungs. This operation allows the patient to swallow food. In both cases, however, the patient is unable to speak without a special assist device.

A ventilator on which the flow rate, inspiratory rate, and inspiratory time may be set is illustrated in Figure 10.6.

VOLUME-CONTROLLED VENTILATOR MODES OF OPERATION

In order to describe the common modes of operation of a volume-controlled ventilator, a simplified microprocessor-based ventilator is shown in Figure 10.7. This diagram consists of several components that need to be described, however, before this figure is discussed.

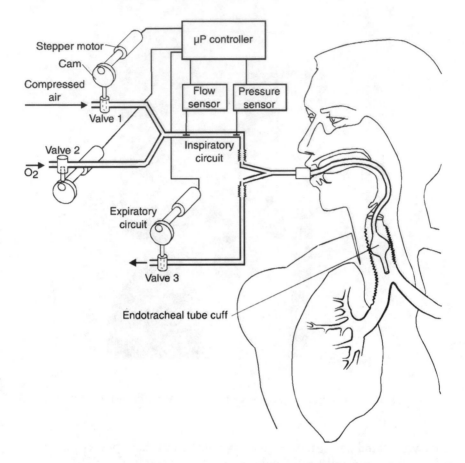

FIGURE 10.7   A simplified ventilator diagram

A *microprocessor* (μP), discussed more fully in Chapter 5, may be defined here as a computer on a chip of silicon one or two square inches in surface area. In this instance, the computer chip is programmed to deliver control voltages of any distribution with respect to time to control a stepper-motor valve (see Spearman).

The *stepper-motor valve* consists of an electric stepper motor, a cam, a valve plunger, and tubing, as illustrated in Figure 10.8. Its purpose is to block or restrict, in a controlled fashion, the air tubes in the ventilator. A stepper-motor shaft will take a fixed position for a particular voltage value on its input leads. Stepper motors are used in many other instruments besides ventilators. For example, they are commonly used in electronic typewriters to position the daisy wheel so that the desired letter is typed on the page when its corresponding letter is struck on the typewriter. In this case, a voltage from the microprocessor in the typewriter, activated by pressing a key, puts the stepper

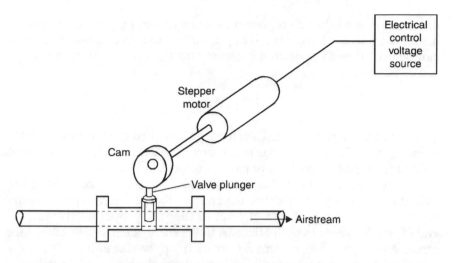

FIGURE 10.8 A stepper-motor valve

motor shaft in the correct position to give the desired letter. In a ventilator application, the stepper motor fixes the cam in a particular posi-
ton for each voltage from the microprocessor control.

The *cam* is an eccentric wheel that pushes the plunger valve into
the air tube as illustrated in Figure 10.9. This diagram shows the cam
pushing the plunger valve into the air tubing as it rotates through three
positions. In the fully open position, the valve is out of the tube so
that it does not restrict the airflow at all. Then rotating counterclockwise, the cam pushes the valve partly into the airstream, restricting
its flow. Again rotating counterclockwise, the cam pushes the valve
further into the tube until the tube is completely closed. This process

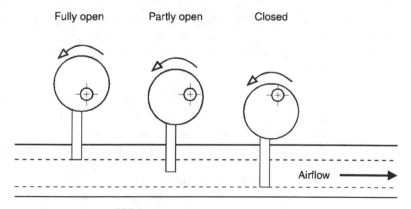

FIGURE 10.9 Valve positions

can continue so that a stepper-motor valve can be placed in several hundred positions between fully open and closed. In this way the valve can be used to set the desired pressure and airflow rate at each instant in the ventilator.

CM Mode

The continuous mandatory (CM) mode (also called the control mode) is the simplest. The ventilator is programmed to deliver a fixed volume of air at a fixed rate, regardless of patient effort.

Following Figure 10.7 again, air and oxygen are taken out of the hospital supply outlet. During the inspiration phase, the μP controls valves 1 and 2 as a function of time so that the proper mixture of air and O_2 are delivered to the patient. A flow sensor, such as a flexible wire strain gauge, in the airstream monitors the flow rate and feeds back a signal to the microprocessor, which regulates the positions of valves 1 and 2 appropriately. During this time, valve 3 on the expiratory circuit is closed so that the air is delivered to the lung of the patient.

During the expiration phase, the μP closes valves 1 and 2 and opens valve 3 so that the patient can release air into the atmosphere.

ACM Mode

The assist/continuous mandatory (ACM) mode delivers a fixed volume of air after the patient makes an effort to breathe. Patient effort sets the timing and rate. This eliminates the feeling of breathlessness that patients frequently experience in the CM mode when they try to breathe spontaneously, but are unable to trigger a flow of air. However, if the patient makes no effort after a preset time, a mandatory breath will be delivered.

To understand the mechanics of this mode, follow Figure 10.7 again. At the end of patient expiration, valves 1, 2, and 3 are closed. Patient effort to inhale produces a negative pressure in the tubing. The pressure sensor triggers the μP, which, in turn, controls valves 1 and 2, to deliver the proper volume and mixture of air and O_2 to the patient. At the end of the inspiratory phase, valves 1 and 2 close and valve 3 opens so that the patient can release the air into the atmosphere. Again, if the patient does not create enough negative pressure through a subsequent inspiratory effort, the breath will be delivered automatically.

IMV Mode

In the intermittent mandatory ventilation (IMV) mode, the patient breathes without assistance, except when an occasional breath is delivered by the ventilator at a preset volume and pressure level. In some cases, the mandatory breath is triggered by patient effort. In other cases, it is independent of patient effort.

To understand how this mode works, follow Figure 10.7. Valves 1 and 2 remain closed and valve 3 remains open while the patient takes several unassisted breaths in and out of valve 3. When it is time for the mandatory breath, all valves close, and patient effort creates a negative pressure in the tubing, which triggers the μP to deliver the breath through valves 1 and 2.

SIMV Mode

The synchronized intermittent mandatory ventilation (SIMV) mode is similar to the IMV mode. In this mode, however, the microprocessor monitors the patient's breathing rate and stores it for reference. Therefore, when a mandatory breath is due, it is delivered to the patient in synchrony with the patient's next breath.

CPAP Mode

Continuous positive airway pressure (CPAP) mode creates a positive pressure from between 5 and 15 cm of H_2O in the patient tubing. The patient breathes unassisted by the ventilator. He or she inhales with the aid of the positive pressure and exhales against that pressure. The effect is to prevent alveolar collapse.

Following the diagram, during inhalation, valves 1 and 2 are set by the μP so that the proper O_2 blend and positive pressure are maintained. During exhalation, valve 3 opens sufficiently so that the patient can exhale against the positive pressure.

PEEP Mode

The positive end-expiratory pressure (PEEP) mode guarantees that a positive pressure in the tubing is maintained throughout both inspiration and expiration. In other words, the exhalation valve 3 will not open until the machine or the patient has created between 5 and 15 cm of H_2O of pressure. The ventilator may then be run in any of the other modes along with PEEP.

For example, creating CM/PEEP with a 10 cm of H_2O end-expiratory pressure would work as described for the CM mode except that valve 3 would not open unless the pressure were above 10 cm of H_2O.

HFPPV Mode

High-frequency positive pressure ventilation (HFPPV) delivers air through a catheter in a cuffed endotracheal tube that may blow air into the lungs at frequencies of 60 to 120 bpm above the normal rate. This allows the maintenance of low mean airway pressures and therefore requires less distension of the lungs. The TV is reduced to keep the alveolar pressure low. The higher air exchange rate compensates for the reduced volume of air so that the patient receives an adequate respiratory oxygen/carbon dioxide exchange.

HFJV Mode

High-frequency jet ventilation (HFJV) consists of the delivery of short pulses of air at a rate higher than the breathing rate of the patient. The air may be delivered through a small-diameter tube inserted through the endotracheal tube. The tube may be uncuffed to leave the airway open. The pulses may be delivered at a rate of 150 pulses per minute (ppm) or more. The effect is to allow the delivery of adequate ventilation at reduced peak airway pressures, thereby reducing stress and possible barotrauma to the patient.

PC-IRV Mode

The pressure-controlled inverse-ratio (PC-IRV) mode of ventilation reverses the conventional inspiratory to expiratory (I:E) ratio and pressure limits mechanical breaths. PC-IRV uses I:E ratios from 1:1 (50% inspiratory time) to 4:1. It is thought a prolonged inspiratory time can improve gas diffusion by the progressive recruitment and stabilization of previously collapsed alveoli. Also, a shortened expiratory time prevents the collapse of alveoli, increasing functional residual capacity and improving oxygenation. Unfortunately, this brief expiratory time can lead to air trapping or intrinsic PEEP (auto-PEEP). Auto-PEEP has the potential to cause barotrauma and reduce cardiac output by decreasing venous return needed for preload through an increase in intrathoracic pressures. The deleterious effects are similar to those seen with PEEP. The reversed I:E ratios cause a feeling of fullness and sometimes extreme discomfort. The patient becomes anxious and restless, which increases the patient's work of breathing and oxygen consumption. Therefore, sedation of the patient is sometimes necessary with PC-IRV ventilation. During conventional volume-controlled ventilation, the tidal volume is accomplished by applying a preset volume for each breath. Therefore, depending on airway resistance and pulmonary compliance, peak airway pressures are variable. During PC-IRV peak inspiratory airway pressure is preset. This causes the tidal volume to vary with each breath. By using PC-IRV, it may be possible to achieve alveolar ventilation at lower peak airway pressures, therefore lessening the risk of barotrauma.

INDICATIONS FOR VENTILATOR USE

Patients require mechanical ventilation when one or both of the following conditions are present: there is ventilatory failure or there is inadequate oxygenation. For adults, the need for mechanical ventilation is defined clinically in terms of the following parameters:

1. A respiratory rate of greater than 40 or less than 10 breaths per minute (bpm). Respiratory rates over 25 breaths per minute increase the work of breathing significantly.

2. A vital capacity of less than two times the tidal volume. If an otherwise normal patient cannot count to 20 rapidly after a deep inspiration and during exhalation, vital capacity is impaired.

3. Inadequate oxygenation is defined clinically as a PO_2 less than 50 mmHg when the patient is receiving a fractional inspired oxygen (FIO_2), that is the concentration of oxygen delivered, that is greater than 60 percent. The level must be measured with arterial blood gasses. Conditions that result in inadequate tissue oxygenation include adult respiratory distress syndrome (ARDS), reactive airway disease (asthma), chronic obstructive pulmonary disease, cardiac arrest, or cardiac failure. Assessing cyanosis as the method of determining hypoxia is not sufficient. Anemic patients will rarely become cyanotic, and polycythemic patients may look cyanotic in the presence of adequate oxygenation. Cyanosis is also affected by the patient's skin color, the room's lighting, or venous vasoconstriction.

4. A PCO_2 greater than 50 mmHg with a pH less than 7.25; this is respiratory acidosis. Respiratory acidosis is caused by alveolar hypoventilation. The causes of alveolar hypoventilation include chronic obstructive lung disease; cardiac failure; acute infections; narcotic, sedative, or anaesthetic depressant effects on the central nervous system's control of ventilation; head injuries that involve or impinge on the brain stem; or spinal cord injuries above the level of C5.

5. A negative inspiratory force of less than 25 cm of water. Patients with chronic obstructive pulmonary disease (COPD) or those with malnutrition, as well as the previously mentioned conditions, may affect this parameter.

Mechanical ventilation is not limited to cases presenting with just these clinical parameters. The patient's underlying disorder may preclude these parameters and require mechanical ventilation for other reasons. Accurate assessment of individual condition always takes precedence when determining the need for mechanical ventilation. For example, patients with COPD have respiratory centers with an insensitivity to high $^PCO_2$. Their drive to breathe is stimulated by a low $^PO_2$. Thus, the patients' work of breathing, the pH, and the negative inspiratory force may need to be evaluated. Trauma patients with chest injuries will normally hyperventilate to compensate for their injury. Even if their respiratory rate is within the acceptable range, it may mean impending ventilatory failure. Patients with neuromuscular conditions, such as Guillain-Barre-Stohl or myasthenia gravis, multiple sclerosis, or poliomyelitis, may exhibit normal parameters. However, if the measurements' trend in TV or VC is decreasing, intubation and mechanical ventilation should be initiated before rapid deterioration takes place. Unconscious patients secondary to drug overdose may experience rapid deterioration of ventilatory abilities as more drug is suddenly absorbed into the intestine. For these reasons, one should intubate before the criteria for mechanical ventilation is met.

The CM mode is indicated for patients with no or minimal ability to make inspiratory effort, or for those who cannot develop the negative pressure necessary to trigger the ventilator. It is used in patients who exhibit respiratory distress syndrome.

The ACM mode is used in patients who have a normal respiratory rhythm but weak muscle action. This mode may cause hyperventilation because the patient is breathing too rapidly.

The IMV mode is used to allow patients to strengthen their respiratory muscles, although this benefit remains questionable, and it is also used to help wean patients from the ventilator. The SIMV mode is used for the same purpose, but it eliminates asynchrony from the breathing pattern.

The CPAP and the PEEP modes are used to keep the airways patent and to prevent alveolar collapse because of pulmonary edema, atelectasis, (collapsed lung) or decreased surfactant from any cause. CPAP levels are usually set between 5 to 15 cm of H_2O. Pressure is continuous throughout the patient's own inspiration and expiration. To use CPAP, the patient must have the ability to initiate his or her own tidal volume and rate. PEEP has the effect of maintaining a positive pressure above atmospheric, which is artificially maintained throughout the expiratory phase only.

The HFPPV and the HFJV modes may be prescribed for patients who need low tidal volumes to reduce stress on the alveoli and other pulmonary structures. PC-IRV is used to support patients with adult respiratory distress syndrome (ARDS) who require high levels of FIO_2 and/or high levels of PEEP to maintain adequate oxygenation. Administration of high levels of FIO_2 greater than 60% for a prolonged period of time may lead to oxygen toxicity. The use of high levels of PEEP greater than 10 cm H_2O may lead to a reduced cardiac output and the development of barotrauma in the form of pneumothorax.

COMPLICATIONS OF MECHANICAL VENTILATION

Complications occur in the classifications of infection, tissue trauma, metabolic imbalances including acid-base, nutritional and electrolyte imbalances, equipment malfunction and maladjustment, machine leakage currents, and psychological trauma to the patient.

Infection

Infection can be transmitted through the hands of the patient or healthcare provider who touches the nasogastric tube or the endotracheal tube. These pathways were illustrated in Figure 10.5. Contamination may enter through the ventilator tubing, nebulizer, or humidifier. The aspiration of stomach contents may contaminate the endotracheal tube; these contents may enter the lung, causing aspiration pneumonia. Elevation of the patient' head, if possible; decompression of the stomach if distention occurs; use of a small-bore feeding tube with continuous feeding; and frequent checks of residual stomach contents to keep them below 75 to 100 cc might help prevent aspiration.

Protection from infection comes by using proper hand-washing technique, sterile gloves, and disinfection techniques. Reduction of infection from the equipment results from removing condensate from the tubing and accessories; allowing no transfer of equipment between patients; disinfecting the tubing, bags, and spirometers; using expiratory gas filters and traps; and changing the patient ventilator tubing every 24 or 48 hours, depending upon hospital regulations.

Proper care of the tracheostomy and ventilator circuits is required not only for prevention of infection, but also for comfort of the patient. Equipment care and cleaning techniques vary, but in general, tracheostomy tubes should be changed every one to two weeks. The frequency may need to be increased if there is a respiratory infection. Removal of the tracheostomy tube is done only after the stoma is well healed and stable.

The goal of tracheostomy site care is to maintain a clean site to prevent infection. Observation for any bleeding, edema, or granulation tissue should occur at the time. The site should be cleaned twice daily using sterile cotton-tipped applicators and an equal mixture of hydrogen peroxide or providone iodine and water. Tracheostomy ties should be changed daily or whenever soiled. Ventilator circuit should be disposable in the inpatient setting. The entire circuit, tubing, and filter should be changed every twenty-four to forty-eight hours.

Tissue Trauma

Barotrauma (a rupture of the alveoli) from high flow pressures or PEEP may occur immediately after initiating mechanical ventilation. The ventilator produces higher intrathoracic pressures by forcing air into the lungs with positive pressure. This is opposite of the normal inspiratory pattern of atmospheric air moving toward lower intrathoracic pressures. The rupture may be exacerbated if the alveoli do not have back support during machine driven inhalation. The rupture may also be exacerbated by pneumonia, sepsis, underlying lung disease, or surgical laceration. Air may collect in the pleural cavity and cause pneumothorax. Signs of pneumothorax include an absence of breath sounds, a sudden or gradual increase in the peak airway pressure, decreased tactile fremitus, a hyperresonant percussion note, subcutaneous emphysema, and, in severe cases, a tracheal shift to the side opposite the side with pneumothorax. The increased thoracic pressure caused by PEEP may also result in elevations in intracranial pressure by causing a decreased cerebral venous return and increased blood volume in the brain. Elevating the head of the bed may facilitate cerebral venous return by gravity.

Low exhaled volume may be a symptom of an endotracheal tube (ETT) cuff leak. The leak can be felt around the mouth, or the patient may be able to make sounds with the vocal cords. The leak can be stopped by reinflating the cuff or replacing it.

The *minimal leak technique* or *minimal occluding volume* is the preferred method for optimal sealing. This is based upon the assumption that during positive pressure ventilation, the tracheal diameter is maximal at the time of inspiration. Thus, if the cuff barely occludes during peak positive pressure inspiration, there will be the least possible pressure on the tracheal mucosa during the expiratory phase, where the diameter is the least. In other words, a minimal leak should be present at the moment in the ventilatory cycle when the tracheal diameter is maximal. Using the minimal occluding volume technique to create an airtight seal will act to avoid undue pressure on the tracheal mucosa and, thus, keep ischemia to a minimum.

Metabolic and Mechanical Imbalances

The airway may become obstructed by bronchospasm, secretions, edema, kinking of the ETT or ventilator tubing. This would trigger a high-pressure alarm (as would water in the tubing), or the patient could "buck" the machine. These troubles are treated by suctioning and straightening the tubing, by applying a bite block, and by giving emotional support to the patient who may be resisting the machine and biting the tubing. In addition to these increases in airway resistance, lung compliance may decrease, thus requiring greater pressure to deliver the prescribed volume of air.

Abnormal blood gas values may result from poor gas exchange and low cardiac output. These are checked by testing arterial blood gasses or by using transcutaneous transducers and oxygen saturation (SaO_2) monitors. Respiratory alkalosis will also occur from either inappropriately high TV or respiratory rate. This can lead to metabolic alkalosis and its serious sequelae.

The HFPPV mode may result in too low an alveolar pressure and allow the alveoli to collapse. Compensation for this may require the introduction of PEEP. High-frequency ventilation often increases the total amount of air passing through bronchial passages. Drying of and injury to the bronchial tubes or trachea could result. Because of the larger volumes of air exchanged, blocking of the expiratory pathway could rather quickly cause hyperexpansion of the lungs and result in injuries.

Oxygen toxicity can occur when FIO_2 above 0.5 (50%) is delivered for more than 24 hours. Parenchymal damage and absorption atelectasis occur. PEEP may be added in order to keep $^PO_2$ above 60 while trying to maintain FIO_2 less than 0.5.

Hemodynamic complications can occur immediately after intubation and the initiation of mechanical ventilation, or at any time during mechanical ventilation. Hemodynamic effects occur due to decreased ventricular filling and decreased venous return because of positive alveolar pressures generated by the ventilator. Keeping the patient hydrated and monitoring hemodynamic parameters, daily weight changes, and intake and output trends will help prevent hemodynamic complications.

Cuff pressures should be measured periodically. In the normal adult, it is reasonable to conclude that pressures on the tracheal wall in excess of 30 mmHg will completely stop arterial–capillary blood flow. Tracheal wall pressures in excess of 18 mmHg will cause venous flow obstruction. Tracheal wall pressures in excess of 5 mmHg will cause lymphatic flow obstruction. Lymphatic flow obstruction will cause edema, venous flow obstruction will cause congestion, and arterial flow obstruction will cause ischemia. The ideal cuff pressure would permit the sealing of the airway during positive pressure ventilation at the lowest possible tracheal wall pressure. If cuff pressures do not exceed 15 mmHg (21 cm of water), arterial and venous flow would be present throughout the ventilatory cycle. If cuff pressures exceed 50 mmHg with a patient on positive pressure, the following events usually occur: (1) within 24 hours, mucosal edema and erythema can be seen with varying degrees of interrupted capillary flow; (2) within 48 hours, there are areas of epithelial ischemia and necrosis; (3) within 72 hours, there are spotty patches of sloughed mucosa, resulting in denuded submucosa and/or cartilage; (4) within 5 days, there is evidence of necrotic cartilage.

The periodic deflation of the cuff at various intervals is less beneficial than previously believed. There is no evidence that periodic deflation restores blood flow to the tracheal mucosa in less than one hour, and certainly not in five minutes or less. Patients on controlled ventilation do not tolerate the deflation, and cardiopulmonary instability may result. The periodic deflation–inflation routine may also cause the therapist and nurse to be less careful in properly reinflating the cuff.

Condensation and fluid in the tubing provides a conductive pathway from the machine into the lungs. These vital areas are near the heart, so leakage currents there could be more hazardous than the same current applied to the surface of the body. Protection from these currents is achieved by inspecting the equipment for leakage currents according to National Fire Protection Association (NFPA) regulations and ensuring that the equipment is grounded.

To avoid attendant-mediated shocks, the attendant should be grounded to dissipate static electricity and wear insulating gloves when handling the patient's tubing. The gloves worn by the attendant protect the patient against both shock and infection.

Psychological Trauma

The psychological trauma can be frightening to the patient who is dependent upon a machine to assist with breathing. Fear and panic can contribute to asynchrony between patient ventilatory effort and the ventilator, causing a decreased tidal volume. The patient needs constant, calm explanations and emotional support. Patients who are hypoxic will try to compensate and hyperventilate, thereby causing asynchrony and decreased deliverable tidal volume. These patients may need neuromuscular blockade and sedatives to assure their minute ventilation remains adequate. If this method is used, the patient must have constant verbal contact to decrease anxiety. Therapeutic touch and/or the use of guided imagery should be employed to decrease fear, anxiety, and pain. The patient is experiencing a total loss of control of basic functions. She or he needs human companionship, compassion, a reassurance of safety, and a caring response from the nurse.

NURSING DIAGNOSES

Respiratory Nursing Diagnoses

Respiratory nursing diagnoses that relate to a patient on mechanical ventilation include ineffective breathing patterns, ineffective airway clearance and impaired gas exchange. Assessment of breathing includes evaluation of the patient's general appearance and level of consciousness and the depth, placement, and security of the endotracheal tube. Adequate chest excursion, equal breath sounds, symmetrical diaphragmatic movement, decreased work of breathing (as evidenced by an adequate minute ventilation and ease of ventilation), and synchrony with the ventilator are all expected outcomes.

Monitoring impaired gas exchange includes correlating arterial blood gases to the patient clinically and in relation to ventilator settings. The outcome goals should be to maintain $^PO_2$ within safe limits and to maintain pH and $^PCO_2$ within the patient's normal limits.

Ineffective airway clearance is assessed by seeing and hearing bubbling secretions in the tubing, the patient's cough, or the rise of peak airway pressure. Because the patient with an artificial airway is not capable of effective coughing, the mobilization of secretions from the trachea must be facilitated by suctioning. Patients with copious secretions require frequent suctioning.

Complications of suctioning include hypoxemia, arrhythmias, hypotension, and lung collapse. Signs of hypoxemia are manifested in heart rate abnormalities, usually tachycardia with or without arrhythmias and bradycardia. Hypoxemia is prevented by pre-hyperoxygenation and post-hyperoxygenation. The most common arrhythmias that occur are premature ventricular beats. These result from hypoxemia with resultant myocardial hypoxia or vagal stimulation secondary to tracheal irritation. Hypotension may result from the profound bradycardia or prolonged coughing during suctioning. Lung collapse may result from the insertion of a large suction catheter into a small-diameter artificial airway; this would result in inadequate space for air to readily entrain around the catheter. Mucosal damage from suctioning is also a very common problem. There is a high incidence of edematous and hemorrhagic mucosal tissue. The use of a vacuum in excess of –120 mmHg exacerbates this process, but even the proper levels of –80 to –120 mmHg do not eliminate the problem.

Patients should be instructed in proper breathing techniques and exercises such as diaphragmatic breathing. Practicing with the patient by helping the patient feel the movement of the diaphragm will enhance the learning of this difficult technique. It will also assist the patient in learning the actual range of motion of the diaphragm and could assist with weaning as well.

Altered Nutrition: Less than Bodily Requirements

Alteration in nutrition is an important nursing diagnosis. A team approach to nutritional evaluation is ideal. Inadequate nutrition can impair muscle function and ventilatory drive, decrease surfactant, and impair the immune system, which leads to increased susceptibility to infection and failure to wean. Patients on mechanical ventilation become malnourished because the oropharyngeal intubation blocks the swallowing mechanism and prevents eating or because the catabolism due to their disease process has eroded the nutritional state. The adverse effects of this include a decreased skeletal muscle mass, including the respiratory muscles. This results in an ineffective cough, impaired ventilatory drive, and inability to wean from the ventilator. A nasogastric tube, as was illustrated in Figure 10.5 may be used to provide feeding for the patient. Enteral feeding has several complications, the most common being aspiration. The use of small-bore flexible feeding tubes with a lumen size of no larger than 8 French greatly decreases the incidence of aspiration pneumonia. The incidence of aspiration also rises markedly when bolus feedings are used. Other complications of enteral feeding include diarrhea related to formula osmolality, fat malabsorption, lactose deficiency, hypoalbuminemia from malabsorption, and the contamination of the feedings.

An alternative to enteral feeding is parenteral nutrition. The use of this method has decreased in light of the complications and because of the growing knowledge that lack of stimulation of the intestinal villi will produce a loss of function of the body's natural absorption properties. Enteral feeding is superior, but if parenteral nutrition is used, a knowledge of the complications is essential. The incidence of pneumothorax from catheter placement has been estimated to range from 1 to 10 percent, whereas other complications range to 22 percent (Civetta, p. 218). Sepsis, metabolic imbalances including hyperosmolar hyperglycemic non-ketotic states, and hepatic abnormalities are well documented.

Immobility

Impaired mobility will lead to self-care deficit, skin breakdown, and social isolation. Not only does muscle atrophy occur from decreased mobility, but devastating psychological consequences occur as well. Social isolation leads to confusion, stress, and ICU psychosis. Studies have documented a significant increase in poor outcome as a result of ICU psychosis. Range of motion and frequent changes in position, especially movement to a chair, will help improve ventilation and circulation to pressure points. Goal setting with the patient in terms of self-performance in activities of daily living and accomplishing simple exercises every two hours will involve the patient in the plan of care and combat the deleterious effects of immobility. As long as the patient is hemodynamically stable, he or she should be assisted with walking. Set outcome goals with the patient, such as an increase in walking time per day as tolerated. Evaluate the patient's ability to perform activities of daily living (ADLs) and his or her willingness to involve the family in the care. Frequent back massage not only increases circulation to prevent breakdown, but also relieves anxiety. Prevention of these compli-cations is the most important goal.

Fluid and Electrolyte Disturbances

Impaired fluid volume needs to be evaluated because of the increased circulating antidiuretic hormone secondary to the positive pressure ven-tilation. Intake, output, and daily weight need to be evaluated according to trends. For example, a gain or loss of one kilogram of body weight is equivalent to a gain or loss of approximately 1,000 cc of water.

Electrolyte imbalances include either excesses or deficits in glu-cose, sodium, potassium, phosphorus, calcium, and magnesium. Mon-itoring serum electrolytes is essential, with intervals varying according to the patient's condition.

Sleep Pattern Disturbances

Sleep pattern disturbances are common in mechanically ventilated pa-tients, especially when they are isolated in an ICU setting. Knowledge of the patient's own sleep pattern history and bedtime rituals will assist the nurse in modifying the environment to enhance sleep. Studies of sleep patterns in ICU patients have shown that sleep is interrupted as much as every 1 minute by disturbances in the environment, such as alarms, assessments, and hospital personnel. This disrupts the normal 20-minute cycle of rapid eye movement (REM) and nonREM sleep. Peo-ple need to cycle frequently over a 6- to 8-hour period in order to obtain adequate sleep. When patterns are disrupted for only 48 hours, psy-chosis can result. Maintaining a dark environment at night and a light environment during the day and monitoring the patient by close ob-servation and by the use of attached electronic devices (so that the nurse does not have to disturb the patient) might increase sleep time and improve outcome.

Altered Role Performance

Disturbances in body image that occur because a person is dependent upon a mechanical ventilator for a basic function cannot be mini-mized. Acknowledge the patient's fears; allow the patient to under-stand and acknowledge those fears in his or her own time. Acknowledgement and acceptance cannot be forced. Understand that disruptive behaviors are a symptom of a body image disturbance. Anger and hostility toward family and health-care providers are also a manifestation of altered self-concept. Evaluate the patient for grief re-action, and if complicated grief is present, professional psychological counseling may be necessary.

Impaired Verbal Communication

Impaired communication not only increases anxiety by frustrating the patient, but prevents expression of needs and ideas. Providing picture and number boards and writing materials will help in the short term. If the patient is stable, a tracheostomy tube with fenestration that allows air to flow past the vocal cords will allow speech. If there is a long-term communication need, speech therapy may need to be instituted. Assist the patient and family in dealing with the frustration of impaired communication.

Anxiety

Anxiety can be relieved in many ways. Allow the patient to verbalize his or her stressors. Allow verbalization of fear of sexual dysfunction, chronicity of the problem, and death. If the patient allows, family members should be included in problem-solving sessions, because they are experiencing the same fears as the patient. Immediate stress reduction techniques that should be employed by the nurse include instructing the patient in guided imagery techniques, muscle contraction relaxation techniques where isolated muscle groups are contracted and relaxed, music therapy, and therapeutic touch. Therapeutic touch has been used in the reduction of both stress and pain.

WEANING FROM A VENTILATOR

A patient on a ventilator begins to adapt to an artificial environment after about 48 hours. The patient may become dependent upon the oxygen-enriched air, and his or her muscles may begin to weaken and atrophy from diminished use and/or nutritional or electrolyte problems. Weaning may take about one day for a healthy patient who has been on ventilation for 48 hours; however, weaning could take weeks if the therapy has been extensive. There is no evidence that one method of weaning is superior to another. Most patients do not require a gradual withdrawal. Certain parameters must be measured to evaluate weaning, but the most important factor in weaning a patient is the clinical appearance of the patient. Methods of weaning include the use of T-piece trials, intermittent modes, and pressure support.

T-piece weaning involves disconnecting the patient from the ventilator and attaching a plastic tubing adaptor to the tracheostomy or endotracheal tube. One end of the tubing connects to humidified oxygen, while the distal end of the tubing extends past the T-piece to act as a reservoir to prevent the entrainment of room air. The FIO_2 delivered via T-piece is higher in order to compensate for an increased oxygen consumption from the physiological and psychological increased work of breathing. The length of time on the T-piece is arbitrary and depends upon the patient's response. All vital signs, TV, and $\dot{V}_E$ should be evaluated every two minutes and then five minutes after initiation of the trial. Intervals on the T-piece gradually lengthen with every trial until extubation.

Use of the continuous positive airway pressure (CPAP) mode in weaning allows the patient to breathe independently while receiving oxygen, humidified air, and positive pressure but while remaining connected to the ventilator. The duration of independent breathing, the assessment of clinical response, and the respiratory parameters are the same as for the T-piece method. With CPAP, the positive airway pressure maintained assists to prevent small-airway collapse. The ventilator will also continue to measure TV, $\dot{V}_E$, and the patient's spontaneous respiratory rate.

Use of one of the less-supportive modes of ventilation, such as SIMV, is another method of weaning. This involves gradually reducing the number of mechanically delivered breaths as the patient gradually increases independence from ventilator breaths. SIMV may be used with a PEEP of less than 5 cm of H_2O in order to maintain oxygenation in patients with a decreased compliance. If the patient is clinically stable on SIMV, she or he may be ready to come off the ventilator. There is no report of evidence that SIMV is superior to T-piece trials in terms of the prevention of muscle atrophy or the success of weaning. However, SIMV may be the choice for a person who is psychologically dependent on the machine in such a way that she or he is fearful of the sudden withdrawal of mechanical support.

Pressure support or pressure variable ventilation augments spontaneous inspiratory effort with a set amount of positive airway pressure (CPAP). The patient controls ventilation, as well as the rate, length, volume, and force of each breath. The patient first generates a negative inspiratory force spontaneously. The ventilator then delivers a variable volume at a controlled pressure and maintains the flow of air at that peak pressure. The work of breathing is decreased because the patient is in control of respiratory rate and minute ventilation. This method of weaning is purely supportive so the patient must have an intact brain stem for the initiation of ventilatory drive.

Before weaning, it is necessary to check the oxygenation, ventilation, and respiratory parameters, vital signs, improve acid-base balance, and correct anemia, electrolyte imbalances, caloric and protein depletion, and fever. The patient's blood pressure and cardiac rhythm should be within the normal limits for the patient. Arrhythmias decrease cardiac output and, therefore, decrease tissue oxygenation. Every attempt should be made to maintain the $^PO_2$ and $^PCO_2$ near the patient's baseline, rather than aiming for a textbook normal. A high fever increases oxygen consumption, and a reduced hemoglobin reduces oxygen transport—both of which compromise tissue oxygenation. General guidelines recommend $^PO_2$ of greater than 60 mmHg or FIO_2 less than 40–50%. PEEP should be less than 5 cm H_2O.

Other factors that must be improved before weaning can take place are acid-base and electrolyte abnormalities, cardiac output, and infection. Psychological factors include readiness to wean and the evaluation of anxiety and ventilator dependence. The fear of death from suffocation is very real. Nutritional support must also include the evaluation of excessive calories from carbohydrates, which increase carbon dioxide production and may contribute to a failure to wean.

Readiness for weaning is further tested by pulmonary function monitoring. The respiratory rate (RR bpm) should normally be between 12 and 24 but less than 30 to 35 spontaneous breaths in some cases. Minute ventilation should be within the normal range because as compliance decreases, the respiratory rate increases and minute ventilation decreases.

The volume of air the patient exhales unassisted in one minute ($\mathring{V}_E$, or the minute ventilation) should be less than 10 liters per minute. This may be determined by observing the number of times the spirometer cycles in one minute. This is then multiplied by the volume of air in the spirometer (TV). The formula is given in Equation (10.3).

To be ready for weaning, the patient should be able to develop a suction of between –20 and –30 cm of H_2O. This is called the *negative inspiratory force* (NIF). Patients with chronic obstructive pulmonary disease (COPD) may not be able to generate an NIF with this much suction. Minus 12 cm of H_2O may be adequate for weaning for this type of patient.

Another test for weaning is to measure $\mathring{V}_E$ when the patient is making a maximum effort to get the highest value. This is called the *maximum voluntary ventilation* (MVV). To measure MVV, instruct the patient to breathe as deeply and as rapidly as possible for one minute. Then measure RR (bpm) and TV and use Equation (10.3) to obtain the MVV value. It should be greater than double $\mathring{V}_E$ to qualify the patient for weaning.

The final test for readiness to wean is to measure vital capacity (VC). To do this, instruct the patient to inhale as deeply as possible and then exhale all the air possible. The spirometer can then be read for the VC value. V_c is defined as the vital capacity per unit weight. It relates to VC by the formula $VC = V_c \times$ weight. To wean, the value should be between 10 and 15 cubic centimeters per unit of body weight.

In summary, the weaning parameters that are obtained from pulmonary function monitoring are listed in Table 10.1.

TABLE 10.1 Pulmonary Weaning Parameters

PARAMETER	VALUE
$\overset{\circ}{V}_E$	Normal 10 l/min
RR (bpm)	12 to 24 bpm
V_T	Greater than 6.6 ml/kg body weight
NIF	-20 to -30 cm of H_2O
MVV	Double $\overset{\circ}{V}_E$
V_C	10 to 15 cc/kg

(Source: B. Handerhan)

EXAMPLE 10.1 You have a 155-pound patient on a ventilator. What should the patient's vital capacity and tidal volume be to qualify for weaning?

Solution To convert pounds to kilograms, recall that 1 lb equals 0.454 kg and that 1 cc equals 1 ml. Therefore, the patient's weight in kilograms is

$$(155 \text{ lb}) \frac{0.454 \text{ kg}}{1 \text{ lb}} = 70.4 \text{ kg}$$

From Table 10.1, the patient's vital capacity required is calculated as at least

$$VC = \text{Weight} \times V_C$$

$$70.4 \text{ kg} \frac{10 \text{ ml}}{\text{kg}} = 704 \text{ ml}$$

Also, the patient's tidal volume should be at least

$$TV = \text{Weight} \times V_T$$

$$70.4 \text{ kg} \frac{6.6 \text{ ml}}{\text{kg}} = 464 \text{ ml}$$

EXAMPLE 10.2 You have measured a tidal volume of 0.5 l on a patient, whose breathing rate is 15 bpm. What is the patient's minute volume?

Solution Using Equation (10.3), the $\overset{\circ}{V}_E$ is calculated as

$$\dot{V}_E = 0.5\ \ell\ \frac{15\ \text{breaths}}{\text{min}} = 7.5\ \ell/\text{min}$$

According to Table 10.1, this minute volume may be too low to begin weaning the patient from the ventilator.

TROUBLESHOOTING

PROBLEM: Audible high-pressure alarm
Possible causes: There is increased airway resistance from secretions, mucous plugs, kinked tubing or the patient biting on an oral tube, bronchospasm, or anything that changes patient compliance or resistance, including pneumothorax, atelectasis, pulmonary edema, right mainstem bronchus intubation, coughing, or anxiety.
ACTION: Check the patient for audible secretions in the airway or any distress that may indicate a plug is blocking the line. Suction as necessary. If the patient is in distress and the cause is not immediately correctable, manually ventilate the patient. Check for bilateral breath sounds and a decrease or absence of tactile fremitus over the pleural air. If there are any absent or unequal breath sounds or expansion, notify the physician of possible pneumothorax, pulmonary edema, or right mainstem bronchus intubation. Provide a bite block. Provide emotional support for the patient.

PROBLEM: Audible low-pressure alarm
Possible causes: Patient is disconnected; there is a leak in the circuit; patient is trying to speak.
ACTION: Reconnect the circuit to the patient. Check the circuit for leaks. Check for leaks in the endotracheal tube cuff. Check for displacement of the tube above the vocal cords, and if this occurs, reposition the tube and obtain immediate assistance. Initiate alternate communication techniques.

PROBLEM: Audible apnea alarm
Possible causes: Patient is not breathing; patient is disconnected; there is an improper sensitivity setting.
ACTION: Check the patient. The rate may be too low, and the patient may be unable to initiate spontaneous ventilation. Reconnect the patient to the circuit if it is disconnected. Check the sensitivity setting.

PROBLEM: Patient unable to trigger assisted breath
Possible causes: Sensitivity is set too low; there is a leak in the patient circuit.
ACTION: Reevaluate the patient and reset the sensitivity according to physician direction. Check the patient circuit for leaks and replace as necessary.

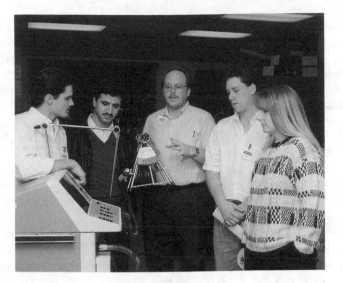

FIGURE 10.10 Testing a ventilator (Courtesy of Johnson City Medical Center Hospital)

An instructor illustrating how to perform tests on a ventilator is shown in Figure 10.10.

REFERENCES

Aston, R. *Principles of Biomedical Instrumentation and Measurement.* Riverside, NJ: Macmillan Publishing Co., 1990.

Carpenito, Lynda J. *Nursing Diagnosis: Application to Clinical Practice.* Philadelphia: J. B. Lippincott Co., 1992.

Civetta, J. M., R. W. Taylor, and R. R. Kirby (eds.). *Critical Care.* Philadelphia: J. B. Lippincott Co., 1989.

Craven, D. E. "Pathogenesis and Prevention of Nosocomial Pneumonia in the Mechanically Ventilated Patient." *Respiratory Care* 34, no. 2 (February 1989): 85–97.

Daronic, G. O. "Ten Perils of Mechanical Ventilation . . . and How to Hold Them in Check." *RN Magazine* (May 1983): 37–42.

Grossbach, I. "Troubleshooting Ventilator and Patient-related Problems, Part 1." *Critical Care Nurse* 6, no. 4 (June 1986): 56–70.

Grossbach, I. "Troubleshooting Ventilator and Patient-related Problems, Part 2." *Critical Care Nurse* 6, no. 5 (June 1986): 64–79.

Guzzetta, C. E., and B. M. Dossey. *Critical Care Nursing: Body-Mind Tapestry.* St. Louis: C.V. Mosby Co., 1984.

Hamilton, L. H. "Ventilators, High-frequency." *Encyclopedia of Medical Devices and Instrumentation.* Vol. 4. Edited by J. G. Webster. New York: John Wiley & Sons, 1988: 2858–64.

Handerhan, B., and N. Allegrezza. "Getting Your Patient off a Ventilator." *RN Magazine* 52, no. 12 (December 1989): 60–66.

Hodgkin, J. E. "Non-ventilator Aspects of Care for Ventilator-assisted Patients." *Respiratory Care* 31, no. 4 (1986): 334–37.

Kenner, C. V., C. E. Guzzetta, and B. M. Dossey. *Critical Care Nursing: Body, Mind and Spirit* (2nd ed.). Boston: Little, Brown & Co., 1985.

Knipper, J. S, and M. A. Alpen. "Ventilatory Support," in G. M. Bulechik and J. C. McCloskey Eds., *Nursing Interventions: Essential Nursing Treatments*. Philadelphia: W. B. Saunders Co., 1992.

Make, B. J. "Long-term Management of Ventilator-assisted Individuals: The Boston University Experience." *Respiratory Care* 31, no. 4 (1986): 303–10.

Marini, J. J. "The Physiological Determinants of Ventilator Dependence." *Respiratory Care* 31, no. 4 (1986): 271–82.

Mayo, J. M., and J. B. Hammer. "A Nurse's Guide to Mechanical Ventilation." *RN Magazine* 50 (August 1987): 18–23.

Prentice, W. S. "Placement Alternatives for Long-term Ventilator Care. *Respiratory Care* 31, no. 4 (1986): 288–93.

Smeltzer, S. C., and B. J. Bane, eds. *Brunner and Sudderth's Textbook of Medical-surgical Nursing*. 7th ed. Philadelphia: J. B. Lippincott Co., 1992.

Spearman, C. B. "The New Generation of Mechanical Ventilators." *Respiratory Care* 32, no. 6 (June 1987): 403–18.

Spearman, C. B. "Positive End-expiratory Pressure: Terminology and Technical Aspects of PEEP Devices and Systems." *Respiratory Care* 33, no. 6 (June 1988): 434–40.

Vasbinder-Dillon, D. "Understanding Mechanical Ventilation." *Critical Care Nurse* 8, no. 7 (October 1988): 42–56.

Whitcomb, M. E. "Care of the Ventilator-dependent Patient: Public Policy Considerations." *Respiratory Care* 31, no. 4 (June 1986): 283–87.

EXERCISES

1. Define a negative pressure ventilator.
2. Define a positive pressure ventilator.
3. Define ventilation.
4. Define respiration.
5. The increase of what gas in the blood increases the respiration rate?
6. The increase of what gas in the blood decreases the respiration rate?
7. Where in the central nervous system is the respiratory control center?

8. Give the definition and the normal value for each of the following pulmonary quantities.

   FRC FVC_1
   VC   TLC
   ERV   MMV
   V_T $\dot{V}_E$

9. Draw the block diagram of a volume-controlled ventilator having pneumatic parts, including an air compressor and bellows.

10. What part of the ventilator in exercise 9 controls the volume of each breath?

11. What mechanism draws the outside air into the ventilator to be delivered to the patient?

12. Describe the bacterial filter and state its purpose.

13. Between the humidifier and nebulizer, which one:
    Uses an aerosol?
    Should be kept at body temperature?
    Delivers medications?
    Uses water?
    Uses an ultrasonic transducer?

14. Using the acronyms in exercise 8, what information would a nurse glean from the spirometer on a ventilator attached to a patient?

15. Define the terms Apnea and Sigh.

16. When the patient has oral intubation, what feeding alternatives are available?

17. Describe two problems a patient with a tracheostomy might experience.

18. Identify the following basic components of a microprocessor-controlled ventilator:

    The position of the shaft can be adjusted by application of a voltage.
    An eccentric wheel
    A computer on a chip

19. What is the relationship between pressure, flow, and airway resistance?

20. Translate the following acronyms:

    CM   SIMV
    PEEP   ACM
    IMV   CPAP
    HFPPV   HFJV

21. In which of the modes in exercise 20 does the patient always breathe at his or her own rate, except when apnea occurs?

22. In which of the modes are breaths always imposed on the patient?

23. Which modes assist in the prevention of atelectasis?

24. Which mode is used when the patient has no ability to make a respiratory effort?

25. In which mode does the patient set his or her own breathing rate?

26. Which mode delivers air at a rate higher than the patient is breathing?

27. Which mode reduces the tidal volume necessary for adequate ventilation?

28. Which mode can be achieved simply by putting a resistance in the exhalation tubing?

29. Name six indications for ventilator use.

30. What are some signs and symptoms of adult respiratory distress syndrome?

31. What are the clinical indications for mechanical ventilation?

32. Name at least 5 classifications of the complications encountered in the patient on mechanical ventilation.

33. To avoid electrical shock, what precautions should an attendant use when handling ventilator tubing?

34. Name three ways that infectious organisms can get to a patient through a ventilator.

35. What accessory in the tubing circuit keeps contamination from the internal parts of the ventilator from entering the patient?

36. How often should ventilator tubing be changed on patients?

37. What physical parameter of the ventilator can cause barotrauma?

38. What can cause pneumothorax in a ventilated patient?

39. What are the symptoms of an ETT cuff leak?

40. How is a leaking ETT cuff corrected?

41. What are three causes of ventilator tube obstruction?

42. Define lung compliance.

43. Why does the peak pressure as set by the ventilator not appear at the alveoli?

44. What mode of ventilation can cause hyperventilation?

45. How long does it take for a patient to adapt to the artificial environment produced by a ventilator?

46. What is the recommended PCO_2 necessary before a patient should be weaned from the ventilator?

47. What is the recommended $^PO_2$ necessary before a patient should be weaned from the ventilator?

48. How do you observe the tidal volume of a patient on a ventilator?

49. If a patient is on the SIMV mode, what mode may be ordered to proceed with the weaning process?

50. List three ventilator modes in the order from the most supportive to the least supportive.

51. You have a 225-lb female on a ventilator. To proceed with weaning, what should be her vital capacity and tidal volume?

Appendix

Voltage and Current Division

VOLTAGE DIVISION

The voltage division principle enables one to determine what voltage appears across a particular element of several connected in series. For example, finding V_{OUT} in Figure A.1 could be done with repeated applications of Ohm's Law. Since the resistors are in series, the current, I may be calculated as

$$I = \frac{18 \text{ V}}{2 \, \Omega + 3 \, \Omega + 4 \, \Omega}$$

$$I = 2 \text{ A}$$

Then notice that I is flowing through R_3 and that V_{OUT} is the voltage it produces across R_3. As required by Ohm's Law,

$$V_{OUT} = (2 \text{ A})(4 \, \Omega) = 8 \text{ V}$$

Because the situation often arises when an attendant is dealing with patient leads where several elements are connected in series, it is useful to memorize a formula for this situation. In Box A.1, it is shown that if three resistor elements are connected in series, that the voltage across one of the resistors is equal to the value of that resistance times the input voltage divided by the sum of the three resistors. The voltage division equation for the variables defined in Figure A.1 is

$$V_{OUT} = \frac{R_3}{R_1 + R_2 + R_3} V_{IN} \tag{A.1}$$

In this case, the circuit has three resistors. A similar formula holds for two resistors, four resistors, or more, so long as they are all in series.

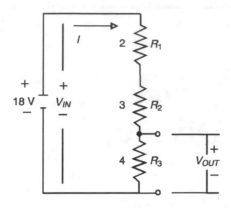

FIGURE A.1　Voltage division

CURRENT DIVISION

In order to determine whether the current flowing down a catheter in contact with a patient's heart exceeds safe limits, the attendant may need to assess how the currents divide among patient leads connected in parallel. In this case, the principle of current division could be used.

As an illustration of this principle, consider the analogy of blood flow. If two blood vessels of equal length were arranged in parallel, and if one had a larger cross-sectional area, it would obviously carry more blood. The one with the larger cross-sectional area would also present less resistance.

In Box A.2, a formula is derived which shows that in the electrical circuit (illustrated in Figure A.2), the current through resistor R_2 in parallel with R_1 will equal R_1 divided by the sum of the resistors R_1 and R_2, and then multiplied by the input current I_{IN}. The formula is

$$I_{OUT} = \frac{R_1}{R_1 + R_2} I_{IN} \qquad (A.2)$$

This equation implies that the larger the resistance in parallel with that carrying the output current, the larger will be I_{OUT}.

EXAMPLE A.2　Using the element and variable values indicated on the circuits in Figure A.3, calculate the output current, I_{OUT}, for part (a) and part (b).

Solution　a. In Figure A.3(a), the input current is 10 A. From Equation (A.2), you can calculate

$$I_{OUT} = \frac{5\ \Omega}{10\ \Omega + 5\ \Omega}\ 10\ A = 3.33\ A$$

_____ BOX A.1 _____

To derive the voltage division equation for Figure A.1, first use Ohm's Law, Equation (1.6), to give the current, I:

$$I = \frac{V_{IN}}{R_1 + R_2 + R_3}$$

Then, Ohm's Law applied to resistor R_3 gives

$$I = \frac{V_{OUT}}{R_3}$$

Equating these two equations gives

$$\frac{V_{OUT}}{R_3} = \frac{V_{IN}}{R_1 + R_2 + R_3}$$

Now, multiplying both sides by R_3 gives the voltage division rule of Equation (A.1).

b. To calculate the current I_{OUT} in Figure A.3 (b), first find the total resistance, R_T in parallel as

$$R_T = \frac{1}{\dfrac{1}{5\,\Omega} + \dfrac{1}{10\,\Omega}} = 3.33\ \Omega$$

this being in parallel with the output resistor. Now I_{OUT} can be calculated from Equation (A.2) as

$$I_{OUT} = \frac{3.3\ \Omega}{2\ \Omega + 3.3\ \Omega}\,5\ A = 3.12\ A$$

NULL CONDITION FOR A WHEATSTONE BRIDGE

To derive the formula that gives the resistor values that cause a null in a Wheatstone bridge, Figure 3.1 should be analyzed. The voltage division principle on the voltage divider on the left of the figure (consisting of R_1 and R_X) yields

_____ BOX A.2 _____

To derive the current division Equation (A.2), write Ohm's Law for V_{IN} in Figure A.2 as

$$V_{IN} = \frac{1}{\dfrac{1}{R_1} + \dfrac{1}{R_2}} I_{IN}$$

Solving for I_{IN}

$$I_{IN} = \left(\frac{1}{R_1} + \frac{1}{R_2} \right) V_{IN}$$

$$= \frac{R_1 + R_2}{R_1 R_2} V_{IN}$$

Ohm's Law applied to Figure A.2 gives

$$V_{IN} = I_{OUT} R_2$$

and this into the previous equation gives

$$I_{IN} = \frac{R_1 + R_2}{R_1} I_{OUT}$$

which when rearranged give the desired Equation (A.2)

$$V_A = \frac{R_1}{R_1 + R_X} V_E$$

Likewise, the voltage divider on the right yields

$$V_B = \frac{R_2}{R_2 + R_3} V_E$$

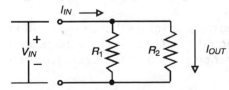

FIGURE A.2   Resistors in parallel

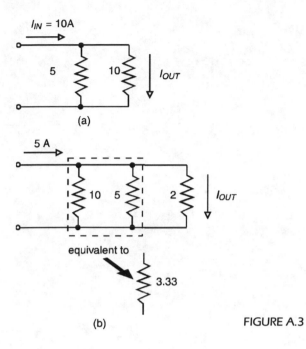

(a)

(b)   FIGURE A.3

The null condition occurs when $V_A = V_B$, making $V_{OUT} = 0$. Under this condition, the equations for V_A and V_B are equal, as the following explanation shows:

$$\frac{R_1}{R_1 + R_X} V_E = \frac{R_2}{R_2 + R_3} V_E$$

Now cancel the V_E on both sides and cross multiply, which gives

$$R_1 R_2 + R_1 R_3 = R_1 R_2 + R_2 R_X$$

Cancelling the $R_1 R_2$ on both sides and dividing by R_2 yields

$$R_X = \frac{R_1}{R_2} R_3$$

which is the same as Equation (3.2) and thus proves the null condition formula.

Index